W9-CYV-813

CONCISE GUIDE TO

Evaluation and Management of Sleep Disorders

Third Edition

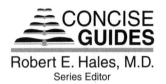

CONCISE GUIDES

Robert E. Hales, M.D.
Series Editor

CONCISE GUIDE TO
Evaluation and Management of Sleep Disorders

Third Edition

Martin Reite, M.D.

Professor, Department of Psychiatry, and
Director, University Insomnia and Sleep Disorders Clinic,
University of Colorado Health Sciences Center, Denver, Colorado

John Ruddy, M.D.

Assistant Clinical Professor, Department of Medicine,
University of Colorado Health Sciences Center;
Staff Physician, National Jewish Medical and Research Center,
Denver, Colorado

Kim Nagel, M.D.

Assistant Clinical Professor, Department of Psychiatry,
University of Colorado Health Sciences Center, Denver, Colorado

American
Psychiatric
Publishing, Inc.

Washington, DC
London, England

Copyright © 2002 American Psychiatric Publishing, Inc.
ALL RIGHTS RESERVED

Manufactured in the United States of America on acid-free paper
06 05 04 03 02   5 4 3 2 1
Third Edition

American Psychiatric Publishing, Inc.
1400 K Street, N.W.
Washington, DC 20005
www.appi.org

Library of Congress Cataloging-in-Publication Data
Reite, Martin.
  Concise guide to evaluation and management of sleep disorders / Martin Reite, John Ruddy, Kim Nagel.-- 3rd ed.
    p. ; cm.
  Includes bibliographical references and index.
  ISBN 1-58562-045-9 (alk. paper)
    1. Sleep disorders--Handbooks, manuals, etc. I. Title: Evaluation and management of sleep disorders. II. Ruddy, John, 1954- III. Nagel, Kim, 1953- IV. Title.
  [DNLM: 1. Sleep Disorders--diagnosis--Handbooks. 2. Sleep Disorders--therapy--Handbooks. WM 34 R379c 2002]
  RC547 .R45 2002
  616.8'498--dc21

                                                                            2001056174

British Library Cataloguing in Publication Data
A CIP record is available from the British Library.

CONTENTS

LIST OF TABLES

5 Parasomnias

6 Medical and Psychiatric Disorders and Sleep

7 Medications With Sedative-Hypnotic Properties

8 Special Problems and Populations

LIST OF FIGURES

INTRODUCTION

to the Concise Guides Series

The Concise Guides Series from American Psychiatric Publishing, Inc., provides, in an accessible format, practical information for psychiatrists, psychiatry residents, and medical students working in a variety of treatment settings, such as inpatient psychiatry units, outpatient clinics, consultation-liaison services, and private office settings. The Concise Guides are meant to complement the more detailed information to be found in lengthier psychiatry texts.

The Concise Guides address topics of special concern to psychiatrists in clinical practice. The books in this series contain a detailed table of contents, along with an index, tables, figures, and other charts for easy access. The books are designed to fit into a lab coat pocket or jacket pocket, which makes them a convenient source of information. References have been limited to those most relevant to the material presented.

Robert E. Hales, M.D., M.B.A.
Series Editor, Concise Guides

ACKNOWLEDGEMENT

The authors could not have produced this volume without the extensive and excellent assistance of Kerri Held McCormick and Linda Greco-Sanders. Their untiring efforts as researchers, editors, proofreaders, and general editorial assistants were greatly appreciated. The assistance of Christy Jones was also greatly appreciated.

OVERVIEW OF SLEEP DISORDERS MEDICINE

Sleep complaints are among the most common voiced by our patients. Not sleeping enough or sleeping too much, experiencing trouble falling or staying asleep, not feeling rested during the day, or having peculiar or annoying things occur during sleep affect almost everyone at one time or another. It is estimated that occasional insomnia occurs in about 27% of the population in the United States, and chronic insomnia in about 9%. Individuals reporting insomnia complain of diminished quality of life—including impaired concentration and memory, decreased ability to accomplish daily tasks, and decreased ability to enjoy interpersonal relationships (Roth and Ancoli-Israel 1999). Untreated insomnia is associated with increases in new-onset anxiety, depression, daytime sleepiness, and other health-related concerns (Richardson 2000). Sleep-related breathing disorders are increasingly recognized as a major cause of morbidity. There appears to be a dose–response relationship between sleep-disordered breathing and subsequent development of hypertension, with its attendant cardiovascular morbidity (Peppard et al. 2000). *The International Classification of Sleep Disorders,* Revised (American Academy of Sleep Medicine 2000) lists in excess of 170 sleep disorders, testimony to the substantial advances in nosology during recent years, yet comprehensive education in the realm of sleep per se (a state in which we spend nearly one-third of our life) or sleep disorders medicine is not yet part of most medical or health care–related curricula.

This volume is designed to provide the practicing clinician with 1) a practical approach to the differential diagnosis and the effective treatment of sleep complaints and disorders and 2) an up-to-date summary of sleep disorders medicine. We emphasize a conceptual framework to facilitate the differential diagnosis, and we include decision trees to facilitate such evaluation. Our goal is to provide access to this rapidly emerging area with sufficient detail to permit the intelligent evaluation and management of most sleep complaints and to indicate where to find information or consultation on the more complex clinical problems. We also hope to help spark an interest in this important area and encourage others to become involved as sleep disorders clinicians and researchers.

■ DIAGNOSTIC NOMENCLATURES FOR SLEEP DISORDERS

Sleep disorders medicine has but recently come of age, and basic nomenclature for sleep disorders varies. Several diagnostic classifications of sleep disorders have been published. The most extensive and detailed classification is *The International Classification of Sleep Disorders,* Revised, published by the American Academy of Sleep Medicine (AASM; http://www.asda.org) (American Academy of Sleep Medicine 2000). This multiaxial classification system has four major categories: 1) dyssomnias; 2) parasomnias; 3) sleep disorders associated with mental, neurological, or other medical disorders; and 4) proposed sleep disorders. This newer classification system replaces the American Sleep Disorders Association's so-called DIMS-DOES-parasomnias classification, first published in 1979 ("Diagnostic Classification of Sleep and Arousal Disorders" 1979), which divided sleep disorders into disorders of initiating and maintaining sleep (DIMS), disorders of excessive sleep (DOES), and the third major area of strange events occurring during sleep, the parasomnias. However, this older "symptom approach" system remains a clinically useful approach to the initial evaluation of a sleep complaint because it captures the manner in which most patients initially present. That is, patients often present with "Doctor, I can't sleep" (the insomnias), "Doctor, I sleep too much" (the excessive sleep disorders), or "Doctor, strange things happen when

I'm asleep" (the parasomnias). In this book, we will emphasize this method of initial approach to a sleep complaint, recognizing that once evaluation is complete, a more specific diagnostic numerical code can be assigned.

DSM-IV-TR, published by the American Psychiatric Association (2000), lists three broad categories of sleep disorders: 1) primary sleep disorders, 2) sleep disorders related to mental disorders, and 3) other sleep disorders. DSM-IV-TR is also a multiaxial classification system, with diagnostic codes compatible with *International Classification of Diseases,* 9th Revision, Clinical Modification (ICD-9-CM; World Health Organization 1995).

ICD-9-CM classifies sleep disorders in three locations: 1) under mental disorders (codes 307.40–307.49), 2) under diseases of the nervous system and sense organs (code 347, narcolepsy), and 3) under symptoms, signs, and ill-defined conditions (codes 780.50–780.59).

This rather confusing system of diagnostic classification will likely prevail until the specific pathophysiologies underlying the various sleep disorders are described, at which time a more specific, and rational, system can be agreed on. Details of these three classification systems can be found in the appendix to this chapter.

■ THE SYMPTOM APPROACH

Sleep disorders medicine has not yet reached the point at which diagnoses can be based on a thorough understanding of the pathophysiological mechanisms involved or on conclusive laboratory studies. Clinicians still depend on the patient to describe his or her symptoms, and these clinicians must obtain a detailed sleep history, a medical workup if indicated, and sleep laboratory studies if indicated to provide corroborative information for the diagnosis.

Typically, patients' complaints fall into the three broad areas described earlier (insomnia, excessive sleep, or parasomnia-type complaints), giving us a starting point in a differential diagnostic evaluation. We must acknowledge that the symptom approach does have certain limitations, however. This approach does not, for example, initially separate true primary sleep disorders from other disorders that affect sleep and result in similar symptoms. For instance, narcolepsy is a true sleep disorder—perhaps specifically a disorder of rapid eye movement (REM) sleep—that results in a set of symptoms that includes excessive daytime sleepiness (EDS). Certain sleep-related breathing disorders (e.g., obstructive apneas), although also presenting as EDS, may not be true sleep disorders; they may actually be disorders of respiratory-related physiology that nonetheless interfere with sleep and thus result in a set of symptoms that includes EDS. Similarly, an insomnia caused by a major affective disorder, which may represent a basic disturbance in the regulation of the function and timing of central nervous system–based sleep systems and thus may be a true sleep disorder, may be grouped with a similarly presenting insomnia resulting from abuse of a sedative-hypnotic or from a sleep-related breathing disorder such as central apnea.

When Should We Consider a Possible Problem?

A common observation in the case of patients with sleep complaints is that they frequently do not seek professional help for the sleep problem per se, or do not mention their problem when seen for other reasons. Studies have shown the incidence of insomnia in primary care to be as high as 69%, yet only one-third of these patients discussed their insomnia with their physicians (Yamashiro and Kryger 1995). Accordingly, it is incumbent on the clinician to raise the issue of possible sleep complaints. The following three questions, which can be covered in about 20 seconds, provide a good initial screen:

1. Are you satisfied with your sleep? (This will suggest most insomnia disorders.)
2. Are you excessively sleepy during the day? (This will suggest most excessive sleep disorders.)
3. Does your bed partner (or parent, in the case of a child) complain about your sleep? (This will suggest a parasomnia disorder).

A positive answer to any of these questions should be reason to consider taking a more detailed sleep history. The sleep history, when performed with the decision trees in mind for the disorder or disorders suspected (for examples of diagnostic decision trees, see Figures 3–1 and 4–1), is the first step in a more comprehensive sleep evaluation. Depending on the outcome of the sleep history, a more detailed differential diagnostic procedure can be tailored to the patient, including perhaps one of the several laboratory studies available for sleep disorders.

Taking a Sleep History

The sleep history involves a careful assessment of the complaint in its medical, environmental, social, and familial context. The following points should be covered:

- When did the symptoms begin, and what has been their pattern since onset? (For example, are they persistent, or do they wax and wane in intensity? Are they seasonal?)
- Were there associated medical-, job-, or stress-related factors at the time of onset? Have these factors persisted, and do they relate to intensity of symptoms?
- What makes the symptoms better? What makes them worse? What happens on a vacation or weekend?
- What is the impact of the sleep complaint on the patient's life?
- What is the patient's typical daily schedule? Is his or her sleep hygiene adequate? (See Chapter 3.)
- Is there a family history of sleep complaints, similar or otherwise?
- What treatments have been prescribed or tried to date, and how effective have they been?
- What medications has the patient used in the past? What drugs are being used currently?

Sources of diagnostic information include the patient, who is usually the one to bring the complaint to the clinician, and others such as the bed partner and other family members or friends. Someone other than the patient with a sleep disorder is often the primary complainant, especially when the patient is a child or when the sleep disorder involves events that occur while the patient is asleep and of which the patient has no memory. In such cases, it is usually quite important to try to obtain such information from another person—either a bed partner (in the case of adult patients) or a parent (in the case of child patients). These observers can provide important information that is usually not known by the patient and that can greatly facilitate diagnostic decision making.

The Sleep Diary

The sleep diary or sleep log (Figure 1–1) can be a most useful adjunct to the history. A detailed and conscientious recording over a 2–3-week period will provide evidence of periodicities often accompanying circadian rhythm disorders, poor sleep related to stressful events, sleep changes in response to medical symptoms or medications, and the like. The sleep diary includes total time in bed (TIB), estimates of time asleep and awake (i.e., all awakenings, time of final awakening, time out of bed), and other factors (e.g., exercise, menstrual periods, meals, activity, drug and alcohol use, and other social events). A completed sleep diary can be used to compute estimates of total sleep time (TST), sleep efficiency (TST/ TIB × 100), number of awakenings during the night, and related numerical indices. These estimates can be used to assess subjective severity and symptomatic improvement.

■ LABORATORY PROCEDURES

Several laboratory procedures are available to assist in the diagnosis of sleep complaints. These procedures include polysomnography, or all-night sleep recordings, and the Multiple Sleep Latency Test (MSLT) to quantify daytime sleepiness (discussed later in this chapter). Additional procedures that might be useful are recording activity 24 hours a day (actigraphy) to quantify circadian activity patterns; recording body temperature 24 hours a day to estimate cir-

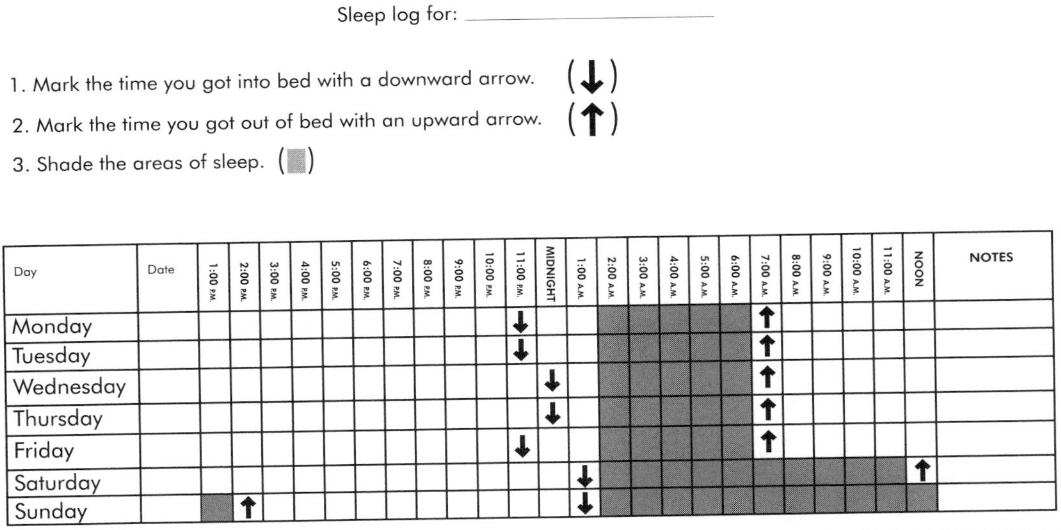

Sleep log for: _____

1. Mark the time you got into bed with a downward arrow. $\left(\begin{array}{c}\downarrow\end{array}\right)$

2. Mark the time you got out of bed with an upward arrow. $\left(\uparrow\right)$

3. Shade the areas of sleep. (▨)

FIGURE 1–1. **Example of a sleep log.**

cadian rhythms; and using the Maintenance of Wakefulness Test (MWT) to quantify the ability to maintain wakefulness. During the MWT, unlike during the MSLT, the patient is in the reclining position and is instructed to try to stay awake. Two protocols (lasting either 20 or 40 minutes) exist.

Advances in technology are permitting some screening laboratory evaluations (e.g., actigraphy, home monitoring for sleep apnea) to take place outside of a formal sleep laboratory environment, which can sometimes be more cost-effective. However, qualified technical support and evaluations must be available in such cases. Furthermore, it is important not to rely completely on simple screening tests such as home oximetry; Yamashiro and Kryger (1995) concluded that home oximetry alone was of limited value as a reliable screening tool for sleep-related breathing disorders.

Polysomnography

Polysomnography entails the recording of multiple physiological variables during sleep. A typical screening polysomnogram (PSG) might include the following variables:

- Electro-oculograms to quantitate horizontal and vertical eye movements
- At least two electroencephalographic channels for sleep staging (e.g., C_3-A_2 and C_4-A_1, and perhaps an occipital lead)
- Chin electromyogram (EMG)
- Left and right anterior tibialis EMGs (separately, if possible)
- Electrocardiogram to measure cardiac rate and rhythm
- Intercostal EMG to ascertain respiratory effort
- Chest and abdominal strain gauges or other systems to measure respiratory excursion
- Nasal and oral thermistors to measure airflow
- Pulse oximetry to measure oxygen saturation

This set of physiological variables permits assessment of sleep stage, respiration, cardiac rate and rhythm, and presence of periodic limb movements of sleep, formerly called nocturnal myoclonus. Patients with possible nocturnal seizures may require an additional 12–20 or more electroencephalographic channels, perhaps with video monitoring. Patients with sleep-related breathing disorders may be studied using additional measurements to provide a greater clarification of respiratory status, including precise measurements of quantified air exchange, esophageal pressure, and expired air CO_2. Patients who are thought to have gastroesophageal reflux may be studied using esophageal pH sensors. Patients with movement disorders may have electromyographic electrodes on multiple muscle groups. Polysomnographic examinations are normally conducted at night, but recordings may be obtained during the day in shift workers. The patient is instructed to report to the laboratory about 1.5 hours before his or her normal bedtime, to give the technician time to apply the necessary electrodes and transducers. The patient then retires, and, after necessary calibrations, the lights are turned off and the patient is allowed to sleep. Recording times may vary, but they typically last about 7.5–8 hours.

Multiple Sleep Latency Test

The MSLT is a test performed in the sleep laboratory that is designed to quantify the nature and degree of daytime sleepiness in patients complaining of EDS (Richardson et al. 1978). The patient is given five 20-minute opportunities to sleep spaced across the day at 2-hour intervals, typically beginning at 10:00 A.M. The patient is polysomnographically monitored with at least an electroencephalogram, an electro-oculogram, and an EMG, so that wakefulness and the various stages of sleep may be defined. The mean sleep latency (MSL) (i.e., the average for all five tests of the time from the beginning of the test to sleep onset) and the presence of REM sleep are noted. Because sleep deprivation can directly lead to EDS and an abnormally short MSL on the MSLT, this test should be performed the day after a nocturnal PSG to ensure that the patient had adequate sleep the preceding night. In addition, because this test should be done while the patient is in a drug-free state, urine should be obtained during the

MSLT for a routine drug screen. Pathological sleepiness is indicated by an MSL of 5 minutes or less. Normal alertness is confirmed by an MSL of greater than 12–13 minutes. The range from 5 to 12 minutes is a gray zone that can represent EDS from a variety of causes. The occurrence of REM sleep within 10 minutes of sleep onset in two or more naps is strongly suggestive of narcolepsy.

A note on sleepiness is in order here. An individual who is not at all sleepy, who has no sleep debt, will have a MSL of 20 minutes on the MSLT—that is, he or she will not go to sleep during any nap opportunity. This is usually seen only in young adolescents. The adult population is mildly sleep deprived (by choice); thus, an adult's MSL will be less than 20 minutes.

Other Laboratory Procedures

A variety of home monitoring equipment and procedures are now available for screening for sleep apnea. These procedures range from simple measurements of oximetry to more extensive recordings with some assessment of respiratory effort, airflow, body position, and TST.

Typically, a technician will go to the patient's home in the evening to apply recording electrodes, set up equipment, and provide patient instruction. The technician will return the next morning to retrieve the equipment and sleep data.

For activity monitoring (actigraphy), the subject wears small electronic devices (actometers) that measure and store movement for periods up to 10 days or more while the patient follows normal day-to-day routines. The memory of the actometer is downloaded into a computer and provides estimates of time spent awake and asleep, sleep periodicity, and circadian sleep–activity rhythms. Estimates of TST obtained with actigraphy compare favorably with those from a PSG, showing agreement greater than 90% in sleep–wake scoring (Sadeh et al. 1994), although sleep morphology or stage information is not available.

Body temperature monitoring for 24 hours a day can often be used to estimate circadian periodicity. Body temperature measurements are cumbersome to obtain, however, because subjects must usually wear a rectal probe, although newer, telemetry-based techniques are being developed. The interpretation of basic circadian temperature rhythms is complicated by "masking" due to temperature increases associated with motor activity, exercise, and so on.

Computerized electroencephalography and evoked potential measures offer the promise of permitting more accurate physiological quantification of basic sleep patterns as well as of the insomnias, but these techniques are still experimental.

Nocturnal Penile Tumescence

Nocturnal penile tumescence (NPT) measures penile erections during REM sleep to help in the differential diagnosis of organic compared with psychogenic impotence. However, erectile impairment can be seen in major depression; thus, an abnormal NPT result is not pathognomonic of organic impotence. Because NPT is primarily a urological diagnostic procedure, it is not discussed further in this volume.

■ SLEEP DISORDERS CENTERS

Sleep disorders centers provide the capability for both diagnostic evaluation and, if desired, consultation and management of most sleep-related complaints. The AASM, a private, nonprofit organization, has designed standards for laboratory assessment of sleep disorders and accredits sleep disorders centers on the basis of evidence that facilities are adequate and that laboratory and clinical personnel are appropriately trained to perform accurate recordings and assessments of sleep disorders. The AASM presently accredits three types of sleep disorders facilities: sleep disorders centers, laboratories for sleep-related breathing disorders, and satellites. A *sleep disorders center* is a medical facility providing clinical diagnostic services and treatment for patients who present with symptoms or features that suggest the presence of any sleep disorder. A *laboratory for sleep-related breathing disorders* provides diagnostic and treatment services limited to sleep-related breathing disorders, such as obstructive sleep apnea syndrome. A *satellite* is a program that is exactly the same as the parent program but in a different location. A satellite cannot be accredited if the parent program is not accredited.

AASM accreditation for sleep disorders centers entails completion of a formal application and a site visit by one or more experienced clinicians to ensure compliance with all requirements. At the time of this writing, there are more than 500 accredited sleep disorders centers and laboratories in the United States.

The American Board of Sleep Medicine (http://www.absm. org) (not yet formally affiliated with the American Board of Medical Specialties) offers a program of certification for physicians and professionals with Ph.D.s, involving completion of a sleep medicine fellowship and passing of both written and oral examinations. Over the past few years, the board has certified between 150 and 200 clinicians per year as specialists in sleep medicine.

How to Use a Sleep Disorders Center

As a rule of thumb, we believe that all patients complaining of EDS should be studied polysomnographically. The exceptions are those cases in which a simple and clear-cut cause is apparent on clinical evaluation (e.g., drug or sedative use or abuse, depression in adolescents, or obvious insufficient sleep), and the EDS resolves with treatment of the underlying cause. In sleep-related breathing disorders, a nocturnal PSG is essential for determining the type and severity of the disorder. We believe that the diagnosis of narcolepsy should be determined with a PSG and MSLT (short MSL with two REM sleep periods within 10 minutes of sleep onset). Even though narcolepsy can be diagnosed in the office on the basis of clinical symptoms (EDS with cataplexy is pathognomonic of narcolepsy), a laboratory evaluation with an MSLT is suggested because people who abuse stimulants can become quite proficient in mimicking the symptoms of narcolepsy to obtain medications. A suspected REM behavior disorder should be accurately diagnosed on the basis of polysomnographic findings (typical increases in electromyographic activity during REM sleep), because the treatment for REM behavior disorders is different from that for other parasomnias. The need for a PSG in other parasomnias (e.g., somnambulism, night terrors) is less well established. If such phenomena are recorded during a videotaped PSG, the diagnosis is clear; however, because their occurrence is sporadic and unpredictable, routine polysomnography is rarely cost-effective in diagnosis.

With the insomnias, when periodic limb movement disorder or central apnea is suspected on clinical grounds, a PSG is required for accurate diagnosis. In other insomnias, PSGs should be limited to patients who are nonresponsive to treatment and for whom the clinician believes additional physiological information will be helpful in diagnosis and treatment planning.

An important question is whether a single night's recording in the sleep disorders center is sufficiently representative of the patient's disorder to result in an accurate diagnosis; that is, how much does sleep disturbance vary from night to night? Researchers have long noted that a "first-night effect" occurs in sleep laboratory recordings. Subjects generally sleep better the second night than the first night, with less time awake, more restful sleep, more REM and Stage III–IV sleep, and possibly shorter REM latencies. Similarly, sleep disturbance may have night-to-night variability (Mosko et al. 1988). Recordings of 2 or 3 nights may be ideal but are generally impractical because of both cost and patient compliance. A single night's recording, to the extent it errs, will likely err in a conservative direction: It may fail to diagnose some (usually borderline) conditions, but it will likely not overdiagnose.

■ REFERENCES

American Academy of Sleep Medicine: The International Classification of Sleep Disorders, Revised: Diagnostic and Coding Manual. Rochester, MN, American Academy of Sleep Medicine, 2000

American Psychiatric Association: Diagnostic and Statistical Manual of Mental Disorders, 4th Edition, Text Revision. Washington, DC, American Psychiatric Association, 2000

Diagnostic classification of sleep and arousal disorders. 1979 first edition. Association of Sleep Disorders Centers and the Association for the Psychophysiological Study of Sleep. Sleep 2:1–154, 1979

Mosko SS, Dickel MJ, Ashorst J: Night to night variability in sleep apnea and sleep-related periodic leg movements in the elderly. Sleep 11:340–348, 1988

Peppard PE, Young T, Palta M, et al: Prospective study of the association between sleep-disordered breathing and hypertension. N Engl J Med 342:1378–1384, 2000

Richardson GS: Managing insomnia in the primary care setting: raising the issues. Sleep 23(suppl):S9–S12, 2000

Richardson GS, Carskadon MA, Flagg W, et al: Excessive daytime sleepiness in man: multiple sleep latency measurement in narcoleptic and control subjects. Electroencephalogr Clin Neurophysiol 45:621–627, 1978

Roth T, Ancoli-Israel S: Daytime consequences and correlates of insomnia in the United States: results of the 1991 National Sleep Foundation Survey II. Sleep 22(suppl):S354–S358, 1999

Sadeh A, Sharkey KM, Carskadon MA: Activity-based sleep-wake identification: an empirical test of methodological issues. Sleep 17:201–207, 1994

World Health Organization: International Classification of Diseases, 9th Revision, Clinical Modification. Salt Lake City, UT, Medicode Publications, 1995

Yamashiro Y, Kryger MH: Nocturnal oximetry: is it a tool for sleep disorders? Sleep 18:167–171, 1995

■ SUGGESTED READINGS

Dement W: The Promise of Sleep. New York, Dell Publishing, 1999

Hauri P, Linde S: No More Sleepless Nights. New York, Wiley, 1996

Hobson JA: Sleep. Scientific American Library. New York, WH Freeman, 1995

Pascualy RA, Soest SW: Snoring and Sleep Apnea, 2nd Edition. New York, Demos Vermande, 1996

Appendix

■ COMPARISON OF INTERNATIONAL
  CLASSIFICATION OF SLEEP DISORDERS,
  DSM-IV-TR, AND ICD-9-CM CLASSIFICATIONS
  OF SLEEP DISORDERS

International Classification of Sleep Disorders

---

1. Dyssomnias

    A.   Intrinsic sleep disorders

1.	Psychophysiological insomnia	307.42–0
2.	Sleep state misperception	307.49–1
3.	Idiopathic insomnia	780.52–7
4.	Narcolepsy	347
5.	Recurrent hypersomnia	780.54–2
6.	Idiopathic hypersomnia	780.54–7
7.	Posttraumatic hypersomnia	780.54–8
8.	Obstructive sleep apnea syndrome	780.53–0
9.	Central sleep apnea syndrome	780.51–0
10.	Central alveolar hypoventilation syndrome	780.51–1
11.	Periodic limb movement disorder	780.52–4
12.	Restless legs syndrome	780.52–5
13.	Intrinsic sleep disorder NOS	780.52–9

    B.   Extrinsic sleep disorders

1.	Inadequate sleep hygiene	307.41–1
2.	Environmental sleep disorder	780.52–6
3.	Altitude insomnia	289.0
4.	Adjustment sleep disorder	307.41–0
5.	Insufficient sleep syndrome	307.49–4
6.	Limit-setting sleep disorder	307.42–4
7.	Sleep-onset association disorder	307.42–5
8.	Food allergy insomnia	780.52–2
9.	Nocturnal eating (drinking) syndrome	780.52–8
10.	Hypnotic-dependent sleep disorder	780.52–0
11.	Stimulant-dependent sleep disorder	780.52–1
12.	Alcohol-dependent sleep disorder	780.52–3
13.	Toxin-induced sleep disorder	780.54–6
14.	Extrinsic sleep disorder NOS	780.52–9

    C.   Circadian rhythm sleep disorders

1.	Time zone change (jet lag) syndrome	307.45–0
2.	Shift work sleep disorder	307.45–1
3.	Irregular sleep–wake pattern	307.45–3
4.	Delayed sleep phase syndrome	780.55–0
5.	Advanced sleep phase syndrome	780.55–1
6.	Non-24-hour sleep–wake disorder	780.55–2
7.	Circadian rhythm sleep disorder NOS	780.55–9

International Classification of Sleep Disorders *(continued)*

---

2. **Parasomnias**
   A. Arousal disorders
      1. Confusional arousals 307.46–2
      2. Sleepwalking 307.46–0
      3. Sleep terrors 307.46–1
   B. Sleep–wake transition disorders
      1. Rhythmic movement disorder 307.3
      2. Sleep starts 307.47–2
      3. Sleep talking 307.47–3
      4. Nocturnal leg cramps 729.82
   C. Parasomnias usually associated with REM sleep
      1. Nightmares 307.47–0
      2. Sleep paralysis 780.56–2
      3. Impaired sleep-related penile erections .. 780.56–3
      4. Sleep-related painful erections 780.56–4
      5. REM sleep–related sinus arrest 780.56–8
      6. REM sleep behavior disorder 780.59–0
   D. Other parasomnias
      1. Sleep bruxism 306.8
      2. Sleep enuresis 788.36–0
      3. Sleep-related abnormal swallowing syndrome .. 780.56–6
      4. Nocturnal paroxysmal dystonia 780.59–1
      5. Sudden unexplained nocturnal death syndrome .. 780.59–3
      6. Primary snoring 786.09
      7. Infant sleep apnea 770.80
      8. Congenital central hypoventilation syndrome .. 770.81
      9. Sudden infant death syndrome 798.0
      10. Benign neonatal sleep myoclonus 780.59–5
      11. Other parasomnia NOS 780.59–9

3. **Sleep disorders associated with mental, neurologic, and other medical disorders**
   A. Associated with mental disorders
      1. Psychoses 292–299
      2. Mood disorders 296, 300, 301, 311
      3. Anxiety disorders 300, 308, 309
      4. Panic disorder 300
      5. Alcoholism 303, 305

International Classification of Sleep Disorders *(continued)*

	B.	Associated with neurological disorders		
		1.	Cerebral degenerative disorders	330–337
		2.	Dementia	331
		3.	Parkinsonism	332–333
		4.	Fatal familial insomnia	337.9
		5.	Sleep-related epilepsy	345
		6.	Electrical status epilepticus of sleep	345.8
		7.	Sleep-related headaches	346
	C.	Associated with other medical disorders		
		1.	Sleeping sickness	086
		2.	Nocturnal cardiac ischemia	411–414
		3.	Chronic obstructive pulmonary disease	490–494
		4.	Sleep-related asthma	493
		5.	Sleep-related gastroesophageal reflux	530.81
		6.	Peptic ulcer disease	531–534
		7.	Fibrositis syndrome	729.1
4.	**Proposed sleep disorders**			
		1.	Short sleeper	307.49–0
		2.	Long sleeper	307.49–2
		3.	Subwakefulness syndrome	307.47–1
		4.	Fragmentary myoclonus	780.59–7
		5.	Sleep hyperhidrosis	780.8
		6.	Menstrual-associated sleep disorder	780.54–3
		7.	Pregnancy-associated sleep disorder	780.59–6
		8.	Terrifying hypnagogic hallucinations	307.47–4
		9.	Sleep-related neurogenic tachypnea	780.53–2
		10.	Sleep-related laryngospasm	780.59–4
		11.	Sleep choking syndrome	307.42–1

Note. NOS=not otherwise specified; REM=rapid eye movement.

DSM-IV-TR Classification of Sleep Disorders

Primary sleep disorders

Dyssomnias

307.42	Primary insomnia
307.44	Primary hypersomnia
	(*Specify if:* recurrent)
347	Narcolepsy
780.59	Breathing-related sleep disorder
307.45	Circadian rhythm sleep disorder
	(*Specify type:* delayed sleep phase type/jet lag type/shift work type/unspecified type)
307.47	Dyssomnia NOS

Parasomnias

307.47	Nightmare disorder
307.46	Sleep terror disorder
307.46	Sleepwalking disorder
307.47	Parasomnia NOS

Sleep disorders related to another mental disorder

307.42	Insomnia related to…
	(*Indicate the Axis I or Axis II disorder*)
307.44	Hypersomnia related to…
	(*Indicate the Axis I or Axis II disorder*)

Other sleep disorders

780.xx	Sleep disorder due to…
	(*Indicate the general medical condition*)
.52	Insomnia type
.54	Hypersomnia type
.59	Parasomnia type
.59	Mixed type
---.--	Substance-induced sleep disorder
	(*refer to substance-related disorders for substance-specific codes*)
	Specify type: insomnia type/hypersomnia type/parasomnia type/mixed type
	Specify if: with onset during intoxication/with onset during withdrawal

---

Note. NOS=not otherwise specified; REM=rapid eye movement.

ICD-9-CM Classification

307.4   Specific disorders of sleep of nonorganic origin

Excludes narcolepsy (347)
   those of unspecified cause (780.50–780.59)

307.40 Nonorganic sleep disorder, unspecified

307.41 Transient disorder of initiating or maintaining sleep

Hyposomnia   associated with

Insomnia   } intermittent emotional

Sleeplessness   reactions or conflicts

307.42 Persistent disorder of initiating or maintaining sleep
Hyposomnia, insomnia, or sleeplessness associated with
- anxiety
- conditioned arousal
- depression (major) (minor)
- psychosis

307.43 Transient disorder of initiating or maintaining wakefulness
Hypersomnia associated with acute or intermittent emotional
   reactions or conflicts

307.44 Persistent disorder of initiating or maintaining wakefulness
Hypersomnia associated with depression (major) (minor)

307.45 Phase-shift disruption of 24-hour sleep-wake cycle
Irregular sleep-wake rhythm, nonorganic origin
Jet lag syndrome
Rapid time-zone change
Shifting sleep-work schedule

307.46 Somnambulism or night terrors

307.47 Other dysfunctions of sleep stages or arousal from sleep
Nightmares
- NOS
- REM-sleep type
Sleep drunkenness

307.48 Repetitive intrusions of sleep
Repetitive intrusion of sleep with
- atypical polysomnographic features
- environmental disturbances
- repeated REM-sleep interruptions

307.49 Other
- "Short-sleeper"
- Subjective insomnia complaint

ICD-9-CM Classification *(continued)*

347	**Cataplexy and narcolepsy**

780.5   Sleep disturbances

Excludes that of nonorganic origin (307.40–307.49)

780.50   Sleep disturbance, unspecified

780.51   Insomnia with sleep apnea

780.52   Other insomnia
- Insomnia NOS

780.53   Hypersomnia with sleep apnea

780.54   Other hypersomnia
- Hypersomnia NOS

780.55   Disruptions of 24-hour sleep–wake cycle
- Inversion of sleep rhythm
- Irregular sleep–wake rhythm NOS
- Non-24-hour sleep–wake rhythm

780.56   Dysfunctions associated with sleep stages or arousal from sleep

780.57   Other and unspecified sleep apnea

780.59   Other

Note.   ICD-9-CM=*International Classification of Diseases,* 9th Revision, Clinical Modification; NOS=not otherwise specified; REM=rapid eye movement.

2

SLEEP PHYSIOLOGY
AND PATHOLOGY

■ SLEEP ARCHITECTURE

Wakefulness and the various sleep stages are determined by characteristic scalp electroencephalogram (EEG) patterns. Wakefulness is normally accompanied by low-voltage, fast scalp-recorded EEGs, with frequencies usually greater than 8 Hz and amplitudes in the vicinity of 50 μV or less. The most prominent electroencephalographic rhythm of quiet relaxed wakefulness is the alpha rhythm, seen over the back of the head when the eyes are closed. Alpha rhythm consists of rhythmical 8–12-Hz activity, usually about 50 μV in amplitude. This rhythm disappears when the eyes are opened (called *alpha blocking*) or during times of visual imagery even with the eyes closed. Alpha frequency rhythms characterize sensory cortical regions during states of relative inactivity. For example, an alpha frequency rhythm may be seen over sensory-motor cortical regions during relaxation, termed the *mu* or *wicket rhythm,* which ceases with contralateral motor activation.

In this section, we compare illustrations of polygraph recordings during wakefulness, including an EEG, an electro-oculogram (eye movement), and an electromyogram (EMG; chin muscle activity), with those of the several sleep stages. Figure 2–1 illustrates an awake record, with prominent alpha activity.

The transition from wakefulness to sleep—normally Stage I non–rapid eye movement (REM) sleep—is indicated by the appearance in the EEG of slower 5–7-Hz theta activity of generally low

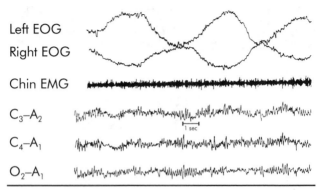

FIGURE 2–1. **Wakefulness.**

This state is characterized by prominent alpha activity in the electroencephalo-gram (EEG), relatively high chin muscle activity in the electromyogram (EMG), and slow rolling eye movements in the electro-oculogram (EOG).

A_1=left ear; A_2=right ear; C_3=left high central EEG; C_4=right high central EEG; O_2=right occipital EEG.

voltage (Figure 2–2). The subject is not responsive at this point but can be easily aroused. Stage I sleep usually constitutes only about 5%–7% of total sleep time (TST).

After a few minutes, the typical subject transitions into Stage II sleep (Figure 2–3), characterized by additional electroencephalo-graphic slowing and the appearance of sleep spindles and K complexes. Spindles are short (usually <1 second) bursts of 12–14-Hz activity dominant over high central regions that wax and wane in amplitude—thus the term *spindle*. They may be generated in, or controlled by activity in, midline thalamic nuclei, such as the centrum medianum. K complexes are large (high-voltage), sharp wave complexes often followed by spindle bursts that are maximally seen over high central and central-parietal regions. They are thought to represent a type of electroencephalographic "evoked response" triggered by external or internal stimuli and may also have deeper brain structures as their source. Stage II is the most common sleep stage, constituting about 50% of total sleep.

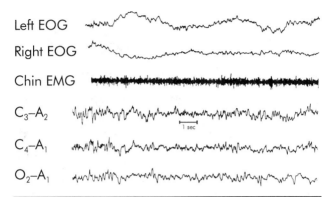

FIGURE 2–2. **Stage I sleep.**

Theta activity predominates in the electroencephalogram (EEG), and there is relatively high chin muscle activity in the electromyogram (EMG) and occasional slow eye movements in the electro-oculogram (EOG).

A_1=left ear; A_2=right ear; C_3=left high central EEG; C_4=right high central EEG; O_2=right occipital EEG.

Stage III and Stage IV sleep usually follow Stage II and are characterized by increased slowing and increased amplitude of the EEG. Stage III sleep contains between 20% and 50% of high-voltage (>75 μV), slow (<2 Hz) delta activity (Figure 2–4), and Stage IV sleep contains more than 50% of slow delta activity (Figure 2–5). Sleep spindles are more difficult to see in Stage III and Stage IV sleep but may still be present. Stage III and Stage IV sleep are often grouped together and termed *delta sleep*. Stage III and Stage IV sleep constitute about 20%–25% of sleep time in adults, but the percentage may be increased in adolescents and decreased in the elderly.

After the typical young adult has been asleep (in non-REM sleep) for approximately 90 minutes, the EEG again transitions to a lower-voltage, faster pattern. The subject remains asleep, but the eyes can now be seen moving beneath the closed lids. Consequently, this stage of sleep is called REM sleep (Figure 2–6). If

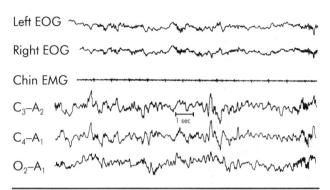

FIGURE 2–3. **Stage II sleep.**

K complexes and sleep spindles appear in the electroencephalogram (EEG). The electromyogram (EMG) is low voltage, and there is electroencephalographic activity in the electro-oculogram (EOG) leads.

A_1=left ear; A_2=right ear; C_3=left high central EEG; C_4=right high central EEG; O_2=right occipital EEG.

awakened during this stage, the subject will often report dreaming. The time from sleep onset (i.e., Stage I) to the onset of the first REM sleep period is termed *REM sleep latency,* which has diagnostic implications. In some psychiatric disorders (e.g., major affective disorders, schizophrenia, and eating disorders), and occasionally in narcolepsy, REM sleep latency is shorter than normal. REM sleep latency tends to decrease with advancing age, but, as a rule of thumb, nocturnal REM sleep latency of less than 60 minutes in an adult should be considered unusually short and might suggest a major affective disorder. REM sleep usually constitutes about 20% of TST in adults.

REM sleep is often described as having *tonic* and *phasic* components. Tonic REM activity consists of the generally low-voltage activated EEG, with a marked decrease in skeletal muscle tone that appears to be mediated by areas near the locus coeruleus. Phasic REM activity includes eye movement bursts, episodic increases in middle ear muscle activity, and episodic electromyographic bursts

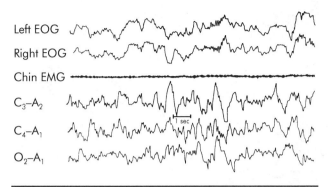

FIGURE 2–4. **Stage III sleep.**

Slow, high-voltage delta activity constitutes 20%–50% of the electroencephalographic activity. There is low chin muscle activity in the electromyogram (EMG), and there is electroencephalographic activity in the electro-oculogram (EOG) leads.

A_1=left ear; A_2=right ear; C_3=left high central electroencephalogram (EEG); C_4=right high central EEG; O_2=right occipital EEG.

(on the generally suppressed electromyographic background). The latter activity has been suggestively correlated with dream content.

REM sleep periods typically end with brief arousals and/or transitions into Stage II sleep again. The completion of the period from Stage I through Stage IV to REM sleep is considered to represent a *sleep cycle,* and a night's sleep (idealized) usually is composed of several (generally around three to five) such consecutive cycles, each about 90 minutes in length.

During a typical night, the nature of the sleep cycles changes considerably. Stage III and Stage IV sleep usually occur only during the first several sleep cycles of the night and usually do not occur during the last sleep cycles. Sleep disorders associated with atypical arousals from Stage III and Stage IV sleep (parasomnias such as sleepwalking and night terrors) tend to occur preferentially early in the sleep period—that is, when most Stage III and Stage IV sleep occur. REM sleep periods (except in patients with depression or a

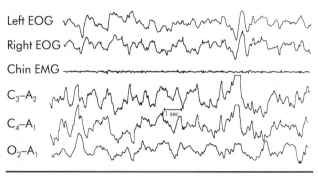

FIGURE 2–5. **Stage IV sleep.**

Slow, high-voltage delta activity constitutes more than 50% of the electroencephalographic activity. There is low chin muscle activity in the electromyogram (EMG), and there is electroencephalographic activity in the electro-oculogram (EOG) leads.

A_1=left ear; A_2=right ear; C_3=left high central electroencephalogram (EEG); C_4=right high central EEG; O_2=right occipital EEG.

major affective disorder) usually are shorter and have fewer eye movements (phasic activity) early in the night and become longer, with more phasic activity and more intense dream activity, as the night progresses. Accordingly, sleep disorders associated with REM sleep (nightmares, REM behavior disorders, and certain sleep-related breathing disorders) may be more pronounced later in the sleep period—that is, when most REM sleep occurs. After a long night's sleep—especially, for example, on a weekend morning when we tend to sleep in—the sleep cycles just before awakening may include only Stage II sleep and REM sleep in equal proportions; therefore, we are likely to awaken from a dream.

■ ONTOGENY OF SLEEP ARCHITECTURE AND SLEEP PATTERNS

Electroencephalographic patterns, sleep morphology, and sleep pattern distribution change dramatically from birth to adulthood. The

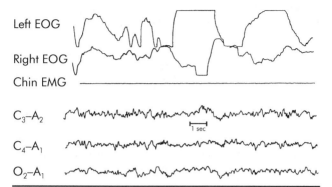

FIGURE 2–6. **Rapid eye movement (REM) sleep.**
This stage is characterized by fast, low-voltage activity in the electroencephalogram (EEG). Chin muscle activity in the electromyogram (EMG) is virtually absent, and there is REM activity in the electro-oculogram (EOG) leads.
A_1=left ear; A_2=right ear; C_3=left high central EEG; C_4=right high central EEG; O_2=right occipital EEG.

newborn, who exhibits a less well organized EEG, spends approximately 50% of sleep time in REM sleep (premature infants spend even more time—up to 80% at 30 weeks' gestational age). This observation, combined with similar data from animal studies, suggests that the REM state is important to early brain development. The REM percentage approaches adult levels (about 20% of TST) during early childhood. Newborns typically have REM onset sleep periods, shifting to adult non-REM onset sleep periods by about age 4 months. Newborn sleep is generally about equally divided into "active" (REM) sleep and "quiet" sleep—the forerunner of later-developing Stage II, Stage III, and Stage IV sleep. At birth, and in premature infants, the EEG of quiet sleep is characterized by a burst-suppression-type or a trace-alternans–type pattern. Stage II and delta (Stage III and Stage IV) sleep can usually be identified by about age 3 months.

TST diminishes with age. It ranges from 16 hours per 24 hours at birth, to about 9 hours at age 6, to about 8 hours at age 12, and typically to about 7.5 hours in adulthood. REM sleep latency in latency-age children is about 2 hours. The first sleep period in late latency and in the early teens usually contains a sustained period of deep Stage III–IV sleep from which it may be quite difficult to awaken the child and during which parasomnias may occur.

During adult life, the percentage of Stage III and Stage IV sleep usually decreases, but this may be primarily because of a decrease in amplitude of electroencephalographic slow waves so that they are no longer formally scorable as Stage III or Stage IV sleep, rather than because of a diminution in an absolute amount of slow-wave electroencephalographic activity. Young adults may spend 25% of sleep time in Stage III and Stage IV sleep; adults at age 50–60 may spend 10% or less of sleep time in these stages. Elderly adults who maintain aerobic fitness may have sustained higher percentages of delta sleep, which are similar to percentages in younger adults. The cyclic nature of normal sleep in a child, a young adult, and an elderly individual is illustrated in Figure 2–7.

In the child, REM sleep latency tends to be prolonged, with an extended amount of Stage IV sleep in the first sleep period. In a young adult, REM sleep latency is about 90 minutes, with little Stage III–IV sleep in later sleep periods. In older adults, sleep is typically more fragmented, with diminished Stage III–IV sleep.

■ BODY PHYSIOLOGY DURING SLEEP

Autonomic activity, such as cardiac and respiratory rate, is usually somewhat diminished and more regular during non-REM sleep than during wakefulness. Skeletal muscle electromyographic activity also diminishes slightly as the sleeping subject relaxes. During REM sleep, however, autonomic activity can become quite variable and highly irregular, with large and rapid changes in cardiac and respiratory rate and blood pressure and prominent activation of peripheral sympathetic autonomic activity (Somers et al. 1993). Most deaths occur in the early morning hours, when the propensity for REM sleep is highest; it has been suggested there may be a relationship between the highly variable physiology accompanying REM and the increased incidence of death in the early morning hours.

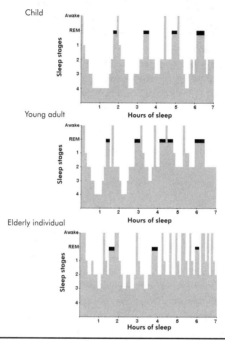

FIGURE 2–7. **Schematic illustration of an all-night sleep histogram in a child (about age 12), a young adult (about age 23), and an elderly individual (about age 70).**

In children, the first sleep cycle contains a great deal of Stage III–IV sleep, which tends to delay rapid eye movement (REM) sleep onset. REM sleep latency may be 2 hours or more. Adults have somewhat less Stage III–IV sleep than children do in the first sleep cycle, with REM sleep latency of about 90 minutes. Elderly individuals have more sleep fragmentation, with increased awakenings, possibly a slightly shorter REM sleep latency, and less Stage III–IV sleep than younger adults (the illustrated hypnogram has no Stage IV sleep).

Body temperature regulation temporarily ceases during REM sleep, and we become for a short time essentially poikilothermic animals. Body temperature also, of course, has a prominent 24-hour "circadian" (about a day) rhythm; temperature tends to be lowest in the very early morning hours and highest in the late afternoon. Sleep is usually associated with a decrease in body temperature, and it is easier to go to sleep when body temperature is decreasing (e.g., in the late evening) and more difficult to go to sleep when body temperature is increasing. REM sleep is most likely to occur when body temperature is lowest, and the peak of REM sleep propensity is coincidental with the initial rising slope of body temperature just after it reaches its lowest point (Czeisler et al. 1980).

REM sleep is also frequently accompanied by penile erections in males and clitoral erections in females.

■ CIRCADIAN PHYSIOLOGY AND SLEEP

Like most living organisms, humans have prominent daily, or circadian, biological rhythms, which have important implications for normal sleep regulation and sleep disorders. The body's major circadian oscillator is located in the suprachiasmatic nucleus (SCN) of the hypothalamus. The SCN can oscillate independently, and animal studies suggest that separate genes control the phase, period, and amplitude of its oscillations. The SCN controls many biological rhythms, including those of body temperature, various hormones, and the sleep–wake cycle—or perhaps more precisely the circadian alerting tendency (sometimes termed Process C, described later in this chapter). That is, the sleep–wake rhythm may actually reflect a circadian tendency to maintain wakefulness rather than promote sleep. This rhythm appears to be coupled to the temperature rhythm, with higher body temperatures being associated with an increased tendency to wakefulness, and vice versa.

The normal sleep–wake rhythm is a 24-hour rhythm that is usually synchronized to the circadian temperature and cortisol rhythm. The sleep–wake rhythm may become desynchronized when the sleep–wake schedule is abruptly changed (e.g., during travel in which time zones are crossed rapidly) with the circadian oscillator remaining on the original schedule. This desynchrony between the attempted sleep–wake schedule in the new time zone and the underlying circadian rhythm is one cause of jet lag.

Human subjects who live in caves or other dimly lit environments without time cues typically adopt a sleep–wake rhythm of approximately 24.2–25 hours (Czeisler et al. 1999). This suggests that the normal free-running circadian period of the sleep–wake rhythm is slightly longer than 24 hours and that this rhythm must be phase-advanced about 12 minutes each day to stay in synchrony with the 24-hour rhythm of the sun. Overall, it appears easier to phase-delay than to phase-advance the body's rhythms, because a phase delay is going in the direction of a free-running rhythm. This has practical implications in the adaptation to a new time zone. A phase delay, as in east to west travel (with a later bedtime), is generally easier and more quickly adjusted to than a phase advance, as in west to east travel (with an earlier bedtime). Some individuals have difficulty advancing their daily rhythm even in a consistent time zone and develop circadian rhythm–based sleep disorders, such as the delayed sleep phase syndrome (see Chapter 3).

We are not born with a well-developed circadian sleep rhythm. As every parent knows, the infant does not have a 24-hour sleep–wake pattern at birth; sleep tends to be randomly interspersed throughout the 24-hour period. A sleep–wake rhythm longer than 24 hours begins to emerge at about age 6 weeks, reflecting the activity of the intrinsic sleep–wake rhythm. In most infants, consolidation of sleep during the night and wakefulness during the day begin to be seen at about age 16 weeks, as the intrinsic sleep–wake rhythm of more than 24 hours becomes "entrained" to the 24-hour period in which we live. This entrainment to a 24-hour sleep–wake rhythm from the initial slower intrinsic rhythm is illustrated in Figure 2–8.

Light is a major synchronizer of circadian rhythms, and it has become apparent that circadian rhythms in humans, as in most other organisms, can be reset by appropriately timed exposure to bright light (Czeisler et al. 1986). The phase-response curve (PRC) plots

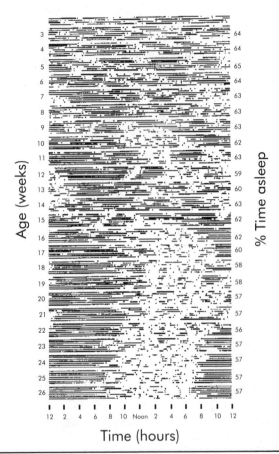

FIGURE 2–8. **Development of the sleep–wake rhythms in human newborn from day 11 to day 182 of life.**

Solid lines represent sleep, *blank areas* represent wakefulness, and *dots* represent feedings.

Source.   Reprinted from Kleitman N, Englemann TG: "Sleep Characteristics of Infants." *Journal of Applied Physiology* 6:269–282, 1953. Used with permission.

how the timing of light exposure affects circadian rhythm timing. The human PRC suggests that exposure to bright light immediately before or shortly after onset of the sleep period (i.e., typically in the late evening) will tend to delay the circadian system, whereas exposure late in the sleep period, shortly before or after awakening (i.e., early morning), will tend to advance the circadian system. Light sensitivity may be related to the time of the lowest body temperature (the nadir of the body temperature circadian rhythm), with light exposure before the body temperature nadir phase delaying the circadian rhythms and light exposure after the nadir phase advancing the circadian rhythms. The human PRC may provide useful information for timing the use of bright-light exposure as a therapeutic modality for treatment of jet lag or circadian rhythm disorders. Therapeutic modifications of the circadian system are covered in Chapter 3. A schematic human PRC to light is shown in Figure 2–9.

Serum cortisol reaches its lowest level around the time of sleep onset and increases before morning awakening, reaching its peak at approximately 8 A.M. This overall pattern of cortisol secretion appears to be circadian in nature and not directly linked to the sleep–wake cycle. Sleep somewhat inhibits cyclic cortisol secretion, and awakenings or sleep fragmentation is associated with increased cortisol secretion during the night. Growth hormone release is generally associated with the onset of Stage III and Stage IV slow-wave sleep in adults. Unlike cortisol, however, growth hormone is locked to the sleep–wake rhythm, and if sleep is delayed, growth hormone is also delayed. Awakenings during Stage III and Stage IV sleep can decrease growth hormone secretion.

Several other hormones have circadian rhythms. Prolactin secretion, like growth hormone secretion, is linked to sleep; prolactin levels increase about 60–90 minutes after sleep onset and peak shortly before awakening. Luteinizing hormone levels increase during sleep in early pubescent subjects but not in adults. This relationship has been used to identify the onset of puberty before secondary sexual characteristics appear.

The hormone melatonin, secreted by the pineal gland at night, appears to influence circadian rhythms. Its secretion is regulated by

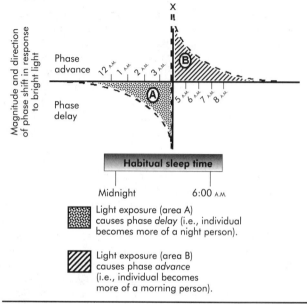

FIGURE 2–9. **Type and magnitude of response of circadian rhythm to bright light exposure.**

Straight line represents time, with the period of habitual sleep indicated at the bottom. *Dashed line* represents the response of the circadian system to bright light, which is minimal during the midday hours. As the night progresses (and body temperature decreases), light exposure progressively delays the circadian system. The effect is reversed at the time of the body temperature's lowest point (nadir); after this point, bright light causes an *advancement* of the circadian rhythm. The maximal response is found shortly before and shortly after the time of core body temperature minimum (X).

light information relayed to the pineal gland from the SCN. Melatonin secretion can be blocked by exposure to bright light during normally dark times. There is emerging evidence that melatonin can be used to reset the circadian system, to treat circadian rhythm disorders, and possibly to treat jet lag and work shift change (Brzezinski 1997). Melatonin generally does not work well as a hypnotic agent. Although the therapeutic use of melatonin is receiving considerable media attention, it has been classified as a food supplement and is available over the counter. Caution should be exercised in terms of its use, as outlined in Chapter 7. Figure 2–10 illustrates the relative timing of several major hormones and body temperature in relation to the sleep–wake cycle.

Process S and Process C

Why do we get sleepy when we do, and why do we awaken when we do? Many investigators suggest a two-process model to explain this—the so-called Process S and Process C model (Borbely and Achermann 1999). Process S is common sense: The longer we have been awake, the sleepier we become. Sleepiness is minimal after a refreshing night's sleep and gradually builds up during time awake.

Process C is essentially independent of Process S and involves the circadian tendency to maintain alertness—maximally expressed in the late afternoon and early evening and minimally expressed in the morning hours (e.g., 3:00–4:00 A.M.). Process C seems to be related to body temperature, which is also maximal in the early afternoon and evening and reaches its lowest point (nadir) about 3:00–4:00 A.M.

The interaction between Process S and Process C is clearly observed when the psychomotor performance of a typical healthy individual is monitored during a short period of sleep deprivation. After a good night's sleep, performance is well maintained throughout the day and the first part of the evening, but there is a prominent decrease in performance after about 17–21 hours of wakefulness. Performance again increases after about 24 hours of wakefulness, even though the subject has remained awake throughout; the circadian wakefulness rhythm boosts alertness (with an associated increase in body temperature) for that next 24-hour cycle. Sleep deprivation–induced psychomotor performance decrements improve after 27 hours of wakefulness, even though no sleep has been obtained.

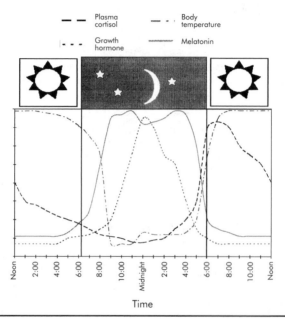

FIGURE 2–10. **Relationship between several circadian rhythms and sleep cycle.**

The time scale of the X axis includes a 24-hour period from noon to noon, with the sleep period represented by the dark (night) section in the middle. Plasma cortisol secretion begins to increase before morning awakening and peaks in the early morning. Growth hormone secretion (which occurs during Stage III–IV sleep) peaks early in the night. Melatonin is secreted after dark and is suppressed by light. Body temperature peaks in the late afternoon to early evening and starts to decrease before sleep onset.

■ NEUROPHYSIOLOGY OF SLEEP

Sleep—both REM and non-REM—is an active process. We do not go to sleep only because of a decrease in sensory input; rather, we go to sleep because of both a decrease in sensory stimulation and an increase in activity of those brain systems that promote the sleep state. Arousal is maintained by the activity of a predominantly cholinergic brain system known as the *ascending reticular activating system* (ARAS). This system is composed predominantly of small neurons with many interconnecting fibers (thus the term *reticular*) that surround the center of the neuraxis, beginning in the spinal cord and ascending into the diencephalon (thus, *ascending*). When the ARAS is electrically stimulated, it arouses or alerts (thus, *activating*) the animal. If the ARAS is lesioned, either experimentally or accidentally, the subject (animal or human) may become somnolent and difficult to arouse. Activity in the ARAS must diminish for sleep to occur. However, in addition, activity in the midbrain raphe and basal forebrain sleep-inducing systems must increase at the same time for sleep (non-REM or slow wave) to ensue and be maintained. Serotonin and γ-aminobutyric acid neurons are involved in slow-wave sleep, as are various peptides, likely including the opiates, α-melanocyte-stimulating hormone, and somatostatin.

REM sleep is also actively triggered by neuronal systems deep in the brain—that is, in the region of the pontine tegmentum. Hobson and McCarley (1977) suggested that gigantocellular tegmental field neurons are influential in this triggering action. Cholinergic mechanisms seem to be important in activating REM sleep systems, and monoaminergic mechanisms are important in interrupting them. These systems may also control the various other manifestations of REM sleep, including eye movements, skeletal muscle postural atonia, general electroencephalographic arousal (low-voltage, fast activity), and unique electroencephalographic waves such as ponto-geniculo-occipital spikes or "sawtooth waves" that accompany REM sleep. The most important issue here is probably that REM sleep is triggered by complex systems deep in the brain stem area that project both up and down and thus control the multiple physiological accompaniments of the REM state. Cholinergic agonists, such as physostigmine, can decrease REM sleep latency in nondepressed adults and can even further decrease REM sleep latency in patients with major depression.

■ DREAMS

The dream is that mental content that frequently accompanies the REM state. Dreams may indeed be "the royal road to the unconscious" in the hands of a psychotherapist, but there is no good evidence for any general form of dream symbolism (such as the snake being a symbol for the penis), and dreams cannot predict the future. Rather, the vivid hallucinatory imagery seems to be a by-product—almost an epiphenomenon—of the heightened state of central nervous system arousal accompanying REM sleep, with the dream perhaps representing the effort of the neocortex to make sense of the essentially random input being received from highly activated lower brain centers (Hobson and McCarley 1977). It remains to be seen whether the specifics of the way in which the neocortex tries to make sense of information in the form of the dream have a predictable and perhaps psychodynamically generalizable form. Dream mentation is not unique to REM sleep; typical dreaming has been reported to accompany other sleep stages as well.

Lucid dreams are dreams in which the dreamer is in the REM state but knows that the dream is a dream—and may even to some extent be able to control the dream. Lucid dreams may occur predominantly during REM sleep with greater-than-normal alpha electroencephalographic content, and some individuals may be able to learn to be "lucid dreamers" (LaBerge 1985).

■ NIGHTMARES

Nightmares are particularly vivid and often anxiety-filled and frightening dreams that arise during REM sleep. Most psychologically healthy adults have one to two nightmares a year, although some individuals have them more frequently. Nightmares tend to decrease in frequency with increasing age but can be increased by stress at any age. They usually do not require treatment per se. Nightmares must be differentiated from night terrors, which are disorders of arousal from non-REM sleep (Hartmann 1984) (see Chapter 5).

■ HUMORAL CONTROL OF SLEEP

Researchers have long been interested in whether some specific factor or substance that triggers or influences sleep may be produced in the brain. Recent research suggests that the purine nucleotide adenosine might be one such sleep factor, perhaps serving as a "final common factor" for previously described putative sleep factors such as interleukin-1 and prostaglandin D_2 (Sinton and McCarley 2000).

■ SLEEP AND IMMUNE FUNCTION

Sleep appears to be closely related to immunological function. The onset of slow-wave sleep specifically has been found to be associated with increases in plasma interleukin-1 activity and with increases in lymphocyte response to mitogen stimulation (Moldofsky et al. 1986). Another peptide, interferon-α, also is involved in immune function. Its level increases during certain viral infections that are accompanied by feelings of depression and malaise, and the peptide has been shown to shorten REM sleep latency (Reite et al. 1987), a phenomenon also associated with major depression in humans.

Sleep deprivation may be accordingly associated with impairment in immune function. Experimental subjects deprived of Stage II sleep have been shown to have decreased natural killer cell activity (Irwin et al. 1994).

■ FUNCTIONS OF SLEEP

Sleep appears to serve a restorative function for the organism. In fact, some investigators have suggested that non-REM sleep serves a restorative function for the body and REM sleep serves a restorative function for the brain. Limited evidence directly supports such theories, with perhaps the best available evidence being that experienced by each person each morning after a good night of sleep. Growth hormone and other anabolic hormones, such as prolactin, testosterone, and luteinizing hormone, have sleep-dependent secretion rhythms, which tends to support the restorative function theory. Other theories consider sleep as a time of energy conservation or postulate that sleep serves an adaptive function in promoting survival. The fact that infants of altricial mammals, including humans, have much more REM sleep at birth than do infants of precocial mammals certainly strengthens the hypothesis that REM sleep supports maturation of the developing brain. The fact that REM sleep can be significantly reduced in adults by injury or by use of REM-suppressing drugs, without apparent ill effects, raises questions about the functions REM sleep serves in the adult brain. Future research must determine which of these various theories of the function of sleep stages can best be empirically supported.

■ SLEEP DEPRIVATION

Animals that are totally deprived of sleep for prolonged periods (up to 30 days) eventually die, with general debilitation and multiple organ failure often initially involving a failure of thermoregulation (Rechtschaffen et al. 1989). Human subjects have tolerated up to about 10 days of acute total sleep deprivation without evidence of serious permanent consequences. Possible long-term physiological effects of chronic mild sleep deprivation such as that experienced by humans in the typical adult population and in most of the chronic insomniac population are unknown. It is clear, however, that substantial adverse effects are related to the increase in sleepiness, which translates to industrial and highway accidents, decreases in job performance, and impaired personal, social, and family functioning. A recent meta-analysis found that sleep deprivation seriously impairs human functioning, with evidence that mood is more strongly affected than either cognitive or motor function (Pilcher and Huffcutt 1996). It has been suggested that as a society, we are chronically mildly sleep deprived either by choice (because of work schedule demands) or as a result of sleep disorders (Bonnet and Arand 1995).

Even short-term sleep deprivation (>24 hours) can impair psychomotor performance. Figure 2–11 demonstrates progressive

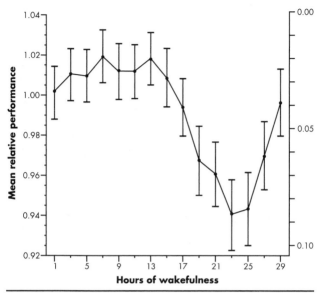

FIGURE 2–11. **Performance in sustained wakefulness condition expressed as mean relative performance and blood alcohol concentration equivalent.**

Error bars represent standard error of the mean.

Source. Reprinted with permission from *Nature* (Dawson D, Reid K: "Fatigue and Alcohol and Performance Impairment" [letter]. *Nature* 338:235, 1997). Copyright (1997) MacMillan Magazines Limited.

decreases in psychomotor performance in healthy adults kept awake for a 28-hour period after a normal night of sleep. In that group, performance began to decrease after 17 hours awake, reaching its low point at 22–24 hours. Then, even though the subjects remained awake, performance began to improve from 27–29 hours, reflecting the activation effects of Process C, the circadian awakening influence. To demonstrate how increasing levels of blood alcohol can similarly decrease performance, researchers subsequently administered increasing amounts of alcohol to the same subject group after the subjects had had a night of normal sleep. Interestingly, the level of performance decrements seen with a blood alcohol concentration of 0.08% (considered legal intoxication in many states) was equivalent to the decrements seen after 24 hours of wakefulness in the absence of alcohol (Dawson and Reid 1997).

■ REFERENCES

Bonnet MH, Arand DL: We are chronically sleep deprived. Sleep 18:908–911, 1995

Borbely AA, Achermann P: Sleep homeostasis and models of sleep regulation. J Biol Rhythms 14:557–568, 1999

Brzezinski A: Melatonin in humans. N Engl J Med 336:186–195, 1997

Czeisler CA, Zimmerman JC, Ronda JM: Timing of REM sleep is coupled to the circadian rhythm of body temperature in man. Sleep 2:329–346, 1980

Czeisler CA, Allan JA, Strogatz SH: Bright light resets the human circadian pacemaker independent of the timing of the sleep-wake cycle. Science 233:667–671, 1986

Czeisler CA, Duffy JF, Shanahan TL, et al: Stability, precision, and near-24-hour period of the human circadian pacemaker. Science 284:2177–2181, 1999

Dawson D, Reid K: Fatigue, alcohol and performance impairment (letter). Nature 388:235, 1997

Hartmann E: The Nightmare. New York, Basic Books, 1984

Hobson JA, McCarley RW: The brain as a dream state generator: an activation-synthesis hypothesis of the dream process. Am J Psychiatry 134:1335–1368, 1977

Irwin M, Mascovich A, Gillin JC, et al: Partial sleep deprivation reduces natural killer cell activity in humans. Psychosom Med 56:493–498, 1994

LaBerge S: Lucid Dreaming. New York, St. Martin's Press, 1985

Moldofsky H, Lue FA, Eisen J: The relationship of interleukin-1 and immune functions to sleep in humans. Psychosom Med 48:309–318, 1986

Pilcher JJ, Huffcutt AI: Effects of sleep deprivation on performance: a meta-analysis. Sleep 19:318–326, 1996

Rechtschaffen A, Bergmann BM, Everson CA: Sleep deprivation in the rat, X: integration and discussion of the findings. Sleep 12:68–87, 1989

Reite M, Laudenslager M, Jones J, et al: Interferon decreases REM latency. Biol Psychiatry 22:104–107, 1987

Sinton CM, McCarley RW: Neuroanatomical and neurophysiological aspects of sleep: basic science and clinical relevance. Semin Clin Neuropsychiatry 5:6–19, 2000

Somers VK, Dyken ME, Mark AL, et al: Sympathetic-nerve activity during sleep in normal subjects. N Engl J Med 328:303–307, 1993

3

INSOMNIA COMPLAINTS

Insomnia is a complaint that can have multiple etiologies, and with the chronic insomnias, more than one cause is quite frequent, necessitating a comprehensive evaluation of every patient. Insomnia complaints are usually grouped into transient insomnias (several days), short-term insomnias (up to 3 weeks), and chronic insomnias (more than 3 weeks).

■ TRANSIENT INSOMNIAS

Transient insomnias (e.g., insomnias of several nights' duration) are ubiquitous. Most individuals experience short-term trouble with sleep latency or sleep maintenance at times of stress, excitement, or anticipation; during an illness; after going to high altitudes; or accompanying sleep time changes (e.g., shift work, jet lag). Such problems rarely come to the attention of the clinician in the early stages, although, of course, clinicians experience these problems themselves. Symptoms of insomnias can nonetheless be decreased, and daytime functioning improved, if certain guidelines are followed. Stress-related insomnia, or temporary trouble sleeping in response to excitement or worry (e.g., when anticipating a trip or a forthcoming interview or examination), may appropriately be treated with a night or two of a short-half-life hypnotic agent (e.g., zolpidem, 5 mg at bedtime). Awakening in the middle of the night with difficulty returning to sleep can be treated with zaleplon 10 mg, so long as the drug is taken no earlier than 4 hours before rising time. The principles of good sleep hygiene (described later in this chapter) are important as well. Pharmacological intervention should be viewed as short term and symptomatic. The appropriate pharmacological treatment of a transient insomnia not only improves daytime performance but also may prevent the insomnia from developing into a chronic problem. There is no reason that responsible patients who know they are susceptible to transient insomnia in relation to predictable stressful events cannot have a hypnotic agent available to use prophylactically as needed.

High-altitude insomnia may occur when individuals rapidly travel to higher altitudes. It frequently accompanies ski and mountain climbing trips. High-altitude insomnia results primarily from altitude-induced periodic breathing with increases in sleep-related central apneas and hypopneas, which can be diminished by several days' administration of acetazolamide (125–250 mg two or three times a day). Acetazolamide also appears to decrease the risk of developing altitude sickness. A short-acting hypnotic such as zolpidem (5–10 mg) or triazolam (0.125–0.25 mg) may also be useful for several nights. Altitude-related insomnia normally improves spontaneously after several days, at least at altitudes below 15,000 feet.

Attempts to sleep at times substantially different from what one is accustomed to—associated with long-distance travel (jet lag) or shift work—often result in disrupted sleep. Treatment (or prevention) of sleep complaints associated with jet lag and shift work is described in the section "Circadian Rhythm–Based Sleep Disorders," later in this chapter.

■ SHORT-TERM INSOMNIAS

Short-term insomnias (up to 3 weeks' duration) are caused by severe and/or persistent stress, such as major surgery, illnesses, or health concerns; significant loss or bereavement; and serious family, job, or relationship problems. The relation of the stress to the insomnia complaint is usually clear. Short-term insomnias should be treated both pharmacologically (short-acting hypnotics) and behaviorally (sleep hygiene, stress management). Bereavement is often associated with a short-term insomnia, which has been reported to respond favorably to sedative tricyclic agents (Pasternak et al. 1994). Untreated short-term insomnias place the individual at risk for a more chronic psychophysiological or conditioned insomnia.

■ CHRONIC INSOMNIAS

The differential diagnosis and effective treatment of chronic insomnia can challenge the most skilled clinician. With chronic insomnias, unlike transient and short-term insomnias, the primary cause is rarely immediately apparent, and the likelihood of more than one cause is significant. We outline a rational, stepwise procedure to facilitate the efficient and accurate differential diagnosis of a chronic insomnia complaint in most patients. Accurate diagnosis is important because different causes of insomnia can present in a similar fashion, and the appropriate treatment for one may aggravate another.

Most patients with chronic insomnia have a presenting complaint of insomnia; however, it is important to realize that a substantial disturbance in nocturnal sleep can present as complaints of chronic fatigue, impaired daytime performance, and excessive daytime sleepiness (EDS), which raises the question of a possible excessive sleepiness disorder. A careful history should identify such patients, however.

A detailed sleep history (see Chapter 1) is the first order of business and should include the type of insomnia problem (sleep onset, sleep maintenance, early awakening), when it began (childhood, recently, at the time of a major stress or life event), when it occurs (every night, weeknights only, at times of stress), what has been done when and by whom, previous response to treatment, whether there is a family history, how the insomnia affects daytime functioning, and similar issues. A sleep diary (see Chapter 1) kept for several weeks may be helpful in establishing the type, perceived severity, and periodicity of the insomnia.

Differential Diagnosis

At this point, the differential diagnosis is facilitated by a systematic approach such as the one outlined here and by using the schematic decision tree in Figure 3–1.

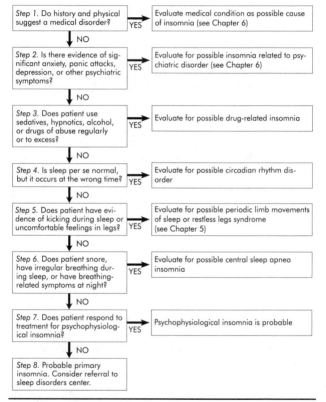

FIGURE 3–1. **Decision tree for differential diagnosis of chronic insomnia.**

Step 1. First, the clinician should inquire about and evaluate the presence of other medical conditions, or treatment for medical conditions, that may contribute to the insomnia complaint. This inquiry may include a complete medical history and, if appropriate, a physical examination with relevant laboratory tests. The clinician should pay special attention to evidence of endocrinopathies and to disorders associated with chronic pain. He or she should keep in mind that the incidence of medical disorders accounting for sleep complaints increases with age. Also, a number of prescription drugs may result in insomnia complaints. A list of commonly used medications that can produce insomnia complaints in some patients is found in Table 3–1. (See Chapter 6 for a more detailed discussion of the relationship between medical disorders and sleep complaints.)

Step 2. The presence of significant anxiety, dysphoric or cyclic mood, or frank depression with sleep complaints should alert the clinician to a possible psychiatric-related insomnia. Nocturnal panic attacks can result in insomnia complaints, even in individuals who do not have typical panic episodes during the day. Accordingly, the clinician should pay special attention to evidence of nocturnal arousals accompanied by autonomic symptoms such as tachycardia, rapid breathing, and the sense of anxiety or fearfulness. Insomnias related to psychiatric causes usually covary with the degree of psychiatric symptoms (see Chapter 6).

TABLE 3–1. **Common drugs with insomnia as a side effect**

β-Blockers	Stimulating tricyclics
Corticosteroids	Stimulants
Adrenocorticotropic hormone	Some selective serotonin reuptake inhibitors
Monoamine oxidase inhibitors	Thyroid hormones
Phenytoin	Oral contraceptives
Calcium-channel blockers	Antimetabolites
α-Methyldopa	Some decongestants
Bronchodilators	Thiazides

Step 3.   A careful drug history will help to identify those patients who have used sedatives or hypnotics, including alcohol, nightly for many months to years in order to fall asleep and who have developed a chronic insomnia secondary to substance abuse. Similarly, a history of stimulant use or drug abuse may result in a sleep disorder. A history of chronic or excessive drug or alcohol use recounted by the patient, or, equally important, by a family member or friend, suggests that further workup in this area is required.

Step 4.   Patients whose sleep is normal (i.e., they go to sleep easily at the right time for them and can sleep uninterrupted and feel rested if they have enough sleep) but whose sleep occurs at the wrong time (e.g., they cannot go to sleep until 4:00 A.M.) may have a circadian rhythm disorder, such as delayed sleep phase syndrome (DSPS). These patients usually present, however, with a chief complaint of insomnia (i.e., "I can't get to sleep until the night is almost over"). The clinician must carefully question these patients to determine whether, once asleep, they are fine if allowed to sleep until they are ready to awaken (e.g., noon) and whether they are chronically sleep deprived if they must rise early for work or school. (The circadian rhythm disorders are discussed later in this chapter.)

Step 5.   The clinician must carefully inquire about the possibility of restless legs syndrome (RLS) or periodic limb movement disorder (PLMD; formerly called nocturnal myoclonus). RLS, characterized by uncomfortable sensations in the calves at sleep onset that require the patient to get up and walk them out, is not a sleep disorder per se but can significantly interfere with the patient's sleep. Periodic limb movements or leg jerks usually are not perceived by the patient (who is asleep) but may be perceived by the bed partner as kicking movements during the night. Patients may say that the bedclothes are in disarray or kicked onto the floor by the morning. Rarely, leg jerks may be noted while the patient is resting in the waking state or napping in a chair. RLS or suspicion of a PLMD requires a more comprehensive sleep workup, including possibly a polysomnogram (PSG) (American Sleep Disorders Association 1995), as detailed later in this chapter (see "Periodic Limb Movement Disorder and Restless Legs Syndrome"). Periodic limb movements may be observed in patients who do not complain of disturbed sleep and who do not arouse from sleep when the leg movements are noted on a PSG. These subjects, although exhibiting leg movements, do not have PLMD.

Step 6. Central apnea is an occasional, albeit uncommon, cause of chronic insomnia, especially in the older patient and at higher altitudes. The clinician should inquire whether the patient has had any subjective sense of trouble getting his or her breath or has been feeling as though his or her breathing is interfered with, especially during the transition from wakefulness to sleep. The clinician should ask the bed partner whether the patient has irregular breathing or pauses in his or her breathing during sleep. Snoring is another clue. Insomnia secondary to sleep apnea is discussed in detail later in this chapter (see "Sleep Apnea Insomnia"). The more common obstructive apneas typically present as EDS (see Chapter 4 for a discussion of these sleep-related breathing disorders).

Step 7. Finally, after the foregoing causes are ruled out, the possibility of primary insomnia, as well as chronic psychophysiological (or conditioned or learned) insomnia, remains. The latter is usually characterized by sleep-onset insomnia that begins during a time of stress and then is aggravated by a fear of not being able to sleep, even after the initial stress has resolved. Patients with this syndrome often sleep better when not in their own beds (e.g., while on vacation) or, paradoxically, in the sleep laboratory, which may result in their symptoms being confused with another cause of chronic insomnia complaints, termed *sleep state misperception syndrome,* in which individuals who appear to sleep normally by conventional electroencephalographic criteria believe that they remain awake.

Step 8. If the patient's condition does not respond to treatment for psychophysiological insomnia, primary insomnia may exist, and a more comprehensive evaluation is indicated, which might include referral to a sleep disorders center.

Clinicians should note that more than one cause of chronic insomnia may be present. A patient may, for example, have a medical, psychiatric, periodic leg movement–related, or other cause of insomnia that has also resulted in a conditioned insomnia component. Many medical problems are complicated by PLMD. Thus, a complete differential diagnosis should be done for each patient; the clinician should not stop when a first probable cause is ascertained.

In the following sections, we will assume that medical and psychiatric histories have been obtained, and we will thus begin with substance use–related insomnia.

■ INSOMNIA OR SLEEP DISTURBANCE SECONDARY TO SUBSTANCE ABUSE, DEPENDENCE, AND WITHDRAWAL

Presenting Complaints

- Poor-quality or nonrestorative sleep in patients dependent on alcohol and hypnotic drugs
- Inability to sleep without alcohol at bedtime
- Severe insomnia for 1–3 days following cessation of sedative-hypnotic or alcohol use
- Persistent insomnia for 2–4 weeks after cessation of alcohol or hypnotic use
- Insomnia after opiate withdrawal
- Sleep-onset insomnia and disrupted sleep in patients who use or abuse stimulants

Drugs and alcohol are used throughout the world for their mind-altering effects. Whether they are used rarely, intermittently, or as part of an abuse or a dependence syndrome, they have the potential to create sleep disturbances such as insomnia, fragmented sleep, hypersomnia, or parasomnias. Many patients seeking treatment for insomnia have a significant component of their condition caused by use or abuse of psychoactive substances. Sleep problems related to drug use occur in both the intoxication and withdrawal phases. Characteristic sleep problems during withdrawal are generally the opposite of those during intoxication (e.g., stimulants induce hypersomnia during withdrawal and insomnia during intoxication), although these problems vary with duration, amount, and regularity of use.

DSM-IV-TR (American Psychiatric Association 2000) includes the category "substance-induced sleep disorder," diagnostic criteria for which are outlined in Table 3–2.

Alcohol

Alcohol-dependent sleep disorder occurs in people who try to self-medicate for a transient or chronic insomnia by using alcohol as a hypnotic. Often these people drink only at bedtime and have no particular interest in alcohol other than for its sedative effects. Usually, the use is minimal, although individual patients may drink more than a pint of hard liquor daily at bedtime to fall asleep. Polysomnography in this group shows that alcohol tends to reduce sleep latency, wakefulness, and rapid eye movement (REM) sleep during the first 3–4 hours of sleep. Later in the night, however, alcohol tends to increase arousals, sleep disruption, sleep fragmentation, and the potential for nightmares because of REM rebound. If possible, these patients should be evaluated for a primary cause of their insomnia and treated. If the clinician does not detect a specific cause, the patient should abruptly stop drinking and use long-acting benzodiazepines at tapering doses to suppress withdrawal symptoms. The initial incident that triggered insomnia may be long gone, and the patient may have continued to use alcohol only to prevent insomnia related to alcohol withdrawal symptoms. If insomnia continues after 4 weeks of sobriety, the clinician should reevaluate the patient to determine the cause of insomnia and treat it appropriately.

Alcohol withdrawal insomnia can be separated into an acute phase (up to 14 days after cessation of alcohol use) and an intermediate and prolonged abstinence phase (several weeks or more after cessation of use). During the early days of withdrawal in alcoholic

TABLE 3–2. **DSM-IV-TR diagnostic criteria for substance-induced sleep disorder**

A. A prominent disturbance in sleep that is sufficiently severe to warrant independent clinical attention.

B. There is evidence from the history, physical examination, or laboratory findings of either (1) or (2):

    (1) the symptoms in Criterion A developed during, or within a month of, Substance Intoxication or Withdrawal

    (2) medication use is etiologically related to the sleep disturbance

C. The disturbance is not better accounted for by a Sleep Disorder that is not substance induced. Evidence that the symptoms are better accounted for by a Sleep Disorder that is not substance induced might include the following: the symptoms precede the onset of the substance use (or medication use); the symptoms persist for a substantial period of time (e.g., about a month) after the cessation of acute withdrawal or severe intoxication or are substantially in excess of what would be expected given the type or amount of the substance used or the duration of use; or there is other evidence that suggests the existence of an independent non-substance-induced Sleep Disorder (e.g., a history of recurrent non-substance-related episodes).

D. The disturbance does not occur exclusively during the course of a delirium.

E. The sleep disturbance causes clinically significant distress or impairment in social, occupational, or other important areas of functioning.

Note: This diagnosis should be made instead of a diagnosis of Substance Intoxication or Substance Withdrawal only when the sleep symptoms are in excess of those usually associated with the intoxication or withdrawal syndrome and when the symptoms are sufficiently severe to warrant independent clinical attention.

    Code [Specific Substance]–Induced Sleep Disorder:

        (291.89 Alcohol; 292.89 Amphetamine; 292.89 Caffeine; 292.89 Cocaine; 292.89 Opioid; 292.89 Sedative, Hypnotic, or Anxiolytic; 292.89 Other [or Unknown] Substance)

TABLE 3–2.   **DSM-IV-TR diagnostic criteria for substance-induced sleep disorder *(continued)***

Specify type:

    Insomnia Type: if the predominant sleep disturbance is insomnia

    Hypersomnia Type: if the predominant sleep disturbance is hypersomnia

    Parasomnia Type: if the predominant sleep disturbance is a Parasomnia

    Mixed Type: if more than one sleep disturbance is present and none predominates

Specify if:

    With Onset During Intoxication: if the criteria are met for Intoxication with the substance and the symptoms develop during the intoxication syndrome

    With Onset During Withdrawal: if criteria are met for Withdrawal from the substance and the symptoms develop during, or shortly after, a withdrawal syndrome

---

patients, sleep is short, fragmented, and light, with virtually no deep sleep and inconsistent changes in REM sleep. If a patient develops delirium tremens, he or she may not sleep at all for several days. Clearly, this period should include vigorous treatment with drugs such as long-acting benzodiazepines to induce sleep and relaxation, reduce seizure potential, and promote physiological stability. Antiepileptic medications, such as phenobarbital or carbamazepine, may also be beneficial for early alcohol withdrawal.

After 2 weeks to 6 months of abstinence, recovering alcoholic patients often complain of insomnia and fatigue and have reduced delta and non-REM sleep, increased arousals and Stage I sleep, increased REM density, and reduced total sleep time (TST). Sleep disturbance has persisted in some patients up to 2 years after withdrawal. Assessment of insomnia in this group can be complex and requires careful consideration.

Overall, the first treatment priority is to begin long-term treatment to maintain abstinence in the alcoholic patient. Concerns about the use of benzodiazepines as sedative-hypnotics to aid sleep beyond the first 4–5 days of withdrawal must be balanced against the greatly increased risk of relapse in abstinent alcoholic patients who continue to have insomnia. Initially, the clinician should encourage sleep hygiene, relaxation, and other nonpharmacological, behavioral means of dealing with insomnia. The clinician should then closely scrutinize this group for affective and anxiety disorders, which have a high comorbidity with substance abuse. Between 2 and 4 weeks of abstinence is a gray area in which many alcoholic patients (or other substance abusers) may have symptoms that fulfill criteria for major depression, bipolar disorder, or an anxiety disorder; however, technically, the 4 weeks needed to allow the diagnosis of a disorder independent of substance abuse have not elapsed. The clinician should consider several strategies in this situation:

- Interview the patient about his or her symptoms present during the last period of abstinence longer than 6 weeks, and use this information to guide treatment.
- Encourage the use of sleep hygiene and behavioral strategies to treat insomnia.
- Use as-needed antihistamines (e.g., diphenhydramine, 25–50 mg, or cyproheptadine, 4–24 mg) when patients are closely monitored but away from their usual sleep environments. The drawbacks are morning grogginess and reinforcement of the need to ingest something to solve problems.
- Treat obvious mania by 2 weeks after alcohol withdrawal; by this time, mania would almost never be mimicked by alcohol withdrawal. Bipolar disorder is common and probably underdiagnosed among substance abusers. More subtle cases can be carefully observed and treated when the diagnosis is clear.
- Be judicious in the use of antidepressants or sedatives during postwithdrawal periods, and be cognizant of the overdose potential of antidepressants (drugs that are resistant to overdose, such as selective serotonin reuptake inhibitors, are recommended) and the high frequency of "occult" bipolar disorders that can be aggravated or unmasked by antidepressants in patients who abuse substances.

- Consider the use of sedative mood stabilizers, such as divalproex, carbamazepine, oxcarbazepine, and gabapentin, which show some promise in offering sedative effects, antikindling effects, no abuse potential, a decrease in irritability, decreased anxiety, and a possible decrease in craving among substance abusers with insomnia related to depressive or bipolar spectrum disorders. Systematic studies are needed to clarify appropriate use in these situations.

Sedative-Hypnotics

Anxiolytics or *sedative-hypnotics* such as benzodiazepines contribute to sleep problems occasionally during use but more frequently during withdrawal or abstinence syndromes. These drugs are very frequently prescribed; more than 1 in 10 Americans use them in an average year. Appropriate use is discussed in Chapter 7.

With regular use of most benzodiazepines, a decrease in Stage III–IV sleep and a moderate suppression of REM sleep would be expected. Although patients may benefit somewhat from nocturnal sedation and reduced anxiety, the lighter-quality sleep and hangover effects of the medications could actually increase daytime fatigue in some people. Some patients interpret this medication-induced daytime fatigue as a need for better sleep. Thus, they may increase their sedative dose in the hope of improved sleep, but they potentially worsen their daytime functioning.

Fatigue related to depression is another example of a symptom that may prompt a person to increase sedative medications to improve sleep, with worsened sleep and restfulness actually resulting. Short- to intermediate-acting benzodiazepines can occasionally cause early-morning awakening or sleep-onset insomnia as a part of withdrawal symptoms that occur even during nightly use. Again, this could unnecessarily lead to continuing or increasing the dose inappropriately.

Patients who continue to have insomnia or daytime fatigue while taking benzodiazepines or other sedative-hypnotics should taper the dose by one therapeutic equivalent per week until they are no longer taking the drug. Then a clinician should reevaluate their insomnia complaints after 2 or more weeks of abstinence.

The most common sleep problem related to benzodiazepine use is insomnia secondary to abstinence or withdrawal syndromes. Three commonly noted problems related to sedative-hypnotic withdrawal are 1) rebound insomnia, 2) moderate drug withdrawal insomnia with reemergence of anxiety or sleepiness, and 3) full-blown and acute drug withdrawal with risk of seizures.

Rebound insomnia is usually associated with abrupt discontinuation of benzodiazepines with short half-lives that have been used at normal doses nightly for a sustained period. This syndrome has been characterized as an increase in difficulty initiating and maintaining sleep for 1–3 days after the abrupt discontinuation of benzodiazepines. It is generally not as severe during withdrawal from longer-half-life sedatives. Rebound insomnia generally can be avoided or attenuated by gradually tapering the sedative dose over 1–2 weeks and by not prescribing higher-than-recommended doses.

Drug withdrawal insomnia is a syndrome that is most classically noted to be associated with abrupt discontinuation of older, multiple-dose nonbenzodiazepine hypnotics (e.g., barbiturates) after prolonged use. Patients report sleep-onset insomnia, fragmented and disrupted sleep, and REM rebound, occasionally with excessive dreaming or disturbing nightmares. Daytime nervousness often increases because of physiological withdrawal, and anxiety intensifies as a result of being without the medication. At times, tremors, dysphoria, diaphoresis, or perceptual abnormalities may occur, depending on how high a drug dose the patient has been taking.

Patients who are undergoing withdrawal from large doses of multiple drugs, as well as alcohol, may experience severe withdrawal symptoms, including anxiety, insomnia, nightmares, grand mal seizures, hyperpyrexia, psychosis, confusion, and even death.

In patients undergoing withdrawal from moderate doses of sedatives, the drugs should be gradually tapered by about one therapeutic equivalent per week. The clinician may want to change the medication to a long-acting benzodiazepine to allow a more comfortable detoxification from ultra-short-acting drugs or from alprazolam (at least when the alprazolam dose reaches 1 mg or less). Doses can be tapered more rapidly for the first 50% reduction, and tapering should be more gradual for the last 50%.

For treatment of withdrawal from high doses of sedative-hypnotics, an inpatient setting may be necessary to manage the potential for delirium, psychosis, or seizures. In addition to prescribing long-acting benzodiazepines, the clinician may consider adding adjunctive medications such as carbamazepine, divalproex, propranolol, clonidine, or phenobarbital.

Opiates

Usually, opiate use and abuse initially affects sleep by reducing TST, sleep efficiency, delta sleep, and REM sleep. Tolerance to these effects usually builds within a week. Opiate users report severe insomnia as part of withdrawal. Often, regular opiate users may alternate between withdrawal states and intoxication states and complain of persistent insomnia without clear knowledge of its relationship to their drug use. Insomnia secondary to opiate use can be diagnosed by history, index of suspicion, and urine drug screens.

Treatment requires confronting the opiate abuse and substituting nonaddictive sedatives. Pharmacological withdrawal strategies include 1) slowly tapering the long-acting opiate (e.g., decreasing methadone by 5 mg/week), 2) adding clonidine to the tapering regimen or increasing clonidine to as high as 0.018 mg/kg/day in three to four divided doses to block autonomic hyperactivity of withdrawal, and 3) administering carbamazepine (200–600 mg/day) to treat sleep problems, irritability, and agitation and, occasionally, to reduce drug craving in patients who still cannot sleep while taking high-dose clonidine or who cannot tolerate the hypotension caused by the full dose of clonidine.

Stimulants

Stimulant-dependent sleep disorder is characterized in the *International Classification of Sleep Disorders*, Revised (ICSD; American Academy of Sleep Medicine 2000) as a "reduction in sleepiness or suppression of sleep by central stimulants, or resultant alteration in wakefulness following drug abstinence" (p. 107). Among the potentially stimulating drugs are amphetamines, methylphenidate, fenfluramine, pemoline, diethylpropion, phentermine, phenylpropanolamine, cocaine, methamphetamine, 3,4-methylene-dioxymethamphetamine (MDMA), propylhexedrine, caffeine, theophylline, ephedrine, and thyroid hormones.

The typical effects of these drugs are to prolong sleep latency and REM sleep latency and to reduce TST and REM sleep time. Tolerance can develop over time in regular stimulant users. During binges of stimulant use, an addicted person may not sleep for days, followed by a day or two of hypersomnolence or "crashing." Many people who abuse stimulants use sedatives to sleep or to regulate the duration or intensity of their high.

Withdrawal from stimulants creates hypersomnia, which is often accompanied by depression and hyperphagia. Sleep studies show increased sleep and REM time with a shortened REM sleep latency. Recognition of the syndrome requires careful history taking, an index of suspicion, and urine drug screenings.

Treatment depends on categorization of use or abuse and on which drug is used:

- Recreational users or stimulant-dependent patients should be confronted with their use and referred to a substance abuse treatment professional. In those with severe withdrawal syndromes (from cocaine or amphetamines), treatment should be supportive and abstinence should be reinforced. In some patients, hypersomnia and depression are so severe during withdrawal that use of desipramine (100–200 mg) may allow an increase in wakefulness and a decrease in depressive symptoms.
- Caffeine users may consider a slow taper of caffeine by one unit (e.g., 1 cup of coffee or soda) every 4–7 days to prevent withdrawal hypersomnolence and headache.
- Patients who require stimulants for attention-deficit disorder or narcolepsy may benefit from changing the timing of the dose, reducing the dose, or switching to slightly less stimulating agents.

- Occasionally, drugs such as theophylline may be necessary to treat a patient's asthma but may be so stimulating that a mild sedative-hypnotic at bedtime is required intermittently or regularly to maintain normal sleep patterns.

Nicotine

Survey data (Phillips and Danner 1995) and polysomnographic studies suggest that cigarette smokers have difficulty going to sleep (increased sleep latency) and problems staying asleep (more wake time). These problems may be caused by nicotine, which has been shown to cause an increase in sleep latency and decreases in both TST and sleep efficiency when given via a transdermal patch to nonsmokers (Davila et al. 1994). Quitting smoking is associated with an acute increase in sleep fragmentation, more frequent arousals and awakenings during the first few days of smoking cessation, and a decrease in daytime alertness as measured by the Multiple Sleep Latency Test (Prosise et al. 1994). Replacement of nicotine via a patch during smoking cessation may ameliorate some of the changes seen during acute tobacco withdrawal (Wetter et al. 1995). Bupropion (Zyban), used as an adjunct during smoking cessation, produces insomnia in nearly one-third of patients treated; adjunctive use of a hypnotic such as zolpidem (5–10 mg) might be considered.

■ CIRCADIAN RHYTHM–BASED SLEEP DISORDERS

Disturbances in the regulation of circadian systems frequently present as sleep complaints. We consider here two general groupings of circadian rhythm–based sleep disorders: *primary* and *secondary*. The first (primary) group includes disorders characterized by a persistent inability to entrain the circadian rhythm of the sleep cycle to that of the rest of the world. These disorders include DSPS, advanced sleep phase syndrome, non-24-hour sleep–wake cycle, and irregular sleep–wake cycle. The second (secondary) group consists of disorders found in persons whose circadian systems may be normal but who are struggling to readjust their circadian rhythms to new situations such as those imposed by work shift change (shift work sleep disorder) or by travel across time zones (jet lag).

Delayed Sleep Phase Syndrome

Presenting complaints

- Sleep-onset insomnia, with difficulty falling asleep until very late at night or early in the morning
- Difficulty awakening in the early morning
- Daytime grogginess and fatigue, especially on days requiring early rising
- Feeling of being alert and energetic late in the evening
- Occasional complaints of depression, especially in adolescents

Clinical presentation.   The typical patient with DSPS may be awake until dawn, trying to fall asleep. Once asleep, the patient will have normal-quality sleep, which will last a normal time unless it is interrupted by the alarm clock or by another external disturbance. The patient may feel well rested on days following a normal sleep period but be sleepy or groggy on days requiring early rising. These patients often become more awake and alert as the day progresses and frequently enjoy working late into the night when others are tired and ready to go to bed. Patients with DSPS are often characterized as night owls. Most adult patients show little sign of anxiety or mood disturbance other than frustration over long sleep latency.

Onset of DSPS in children and adolescents is associated with difficulty getting out of bed in the morning, falling asleep in school, and impaired school performance, often initially interpreted as laziness.

Incidence.   Circadian rhythm–based sleep disorders, especially DSPS, are relatively common. Age of onset is usually adolescence to early adulthood. Many individuals with DSPS may adjust work and activity patterns around their circadian rhythm–based sleep problem—for example, by selecting evening shift work or by doing work that does not require early rising—and never seek treatment.

In children, DSPS may be one of the more common causes of sleep disturbances (e.g., "I don't want to go to bed—I'm not tired," followed by "I can't get up—I'm too tired"). (For discussion of this syndrome in children, see Chapter 8.)

Etiology and pathophysiology.   (See Chapter 2.) The basic period of circadian rhythms and, possibly, their entrainability are likely heritable traits. Persons with DSPS may have a relative inability to phase-advance their circadian rhythms. Melatonin rhythms have been shown to be phase delayed in DSPS (Shibui et al. 1999). In families in which one parent has DSPS, one or more children will also often have a similar sleep tendency. Some data suggest that adolescents may have a normal physiological delay in their sleep rhythm, which results in their common preference to stay up late and sleep late (Carskadon et al. 1993). DSPS has also been described following head trauma (Quinto et al. 2000).

Poor sleep hygiene, such as voluntarily staying up excessively late and sleeping late in the morning, can produce a syndrome that appears to be DSPS. A DSPS-like syndrome may result from psychological causes in persons who use atypical sleep habits to avoid socialization (i.e., to avoid severely stressful events).

Laboratory findings.   Conventional polysomnography is usually not necessary or particularly helpful in evaluation and treatment of DSPS. When these patients are studied in the sleep laboratory, they show prolonged sleep latency, followed by polysomnographically normal sleep, with delayed awakening until the sleep need has been met.

Recording of the circadian temperature rhythm may show a phase delay in DSPS, which can be a useful clue (Ozaki et al. 1988). Masking of the intrinsic temperature rhythm by motor activity can confuse interpretation of temperature recordings, however. Melatonin rhythms may also demonstrate phase delay in DSPS.

Differential diagnosis.   A presumptive diagnosis can usually be made on the basis of history. A sleep diary kept for a 2-week period can be of considerable help. Patients will typically sleep unusually late on weekends or holidays to attempt to recoup the sleep lost during the week, when they must rise early. A record will often show that daytime sleepiness gradually increases as the week progresses. DSM-IV-TR criteria for circadian rhythm sleep disorder are listed in Table 3–3.

The clinician should ask what sleep cycle the patient would choose if he or she could vacation on a tropical island where he or she had no responsibilities. If the patient responds that he or she would go to bed at 4:00 A.M. and rise at noon, this strongly suggests DSPS. The most common mimic of DSPS is poor sleep hygiene, with an intraweek circadian desynchronization. Many people rise much earlier during the workweek than during the weekend. Because of the sleep rhythm's ease in adapting to phase delay, it is easy to sleep until 10:00 A.M. or even later on weekends. When a person sleeps very late on Sunday morning, it may not be until 2:00 or 3:00 A.M. the next night that he or she will have the urge to fall asleep, and secondary tiredness and the tendency to oversleep on Monday morning will result. Establishing a rigorous morning rising time, including on weekends, for a period of 2–3 weeks will usually correct this problem. If this schedule does not help, the clinician should suspect DSPS.

The clinician must carefully screen the patient for affective and anxiety disorders to ensure that the difficulty in rising in the morning is not an aspect of depression (i.e., a tendency for mood to be worse in the morning) or a means to avoid morning family interactions that produce anxiety.

Adolescents with DSPS may have associated symptoms of depression, loneliness, isolation, poor family and peer relationships, and poor school performance. Many of these symptoms may resolve with appropriate treatment of the phase delay.

Treatment.   The treatment of the intraweek circadian desynchronization problem and not true DSPS is good sleep hygiene—that is, strict adherence to constant arousal times 7 days per week, with no more than 1-hour variability from weekdays to weekends. An initial attempt at maintaining good sleep hygiene is usually advisable even

TABLE 3–3. **DSM-IV-TR diagnostic criteria for circadian rhythm sleep disorder**

A. A persistent or recurrent pattern of sleep disruption leading to excessive sleepiness or insomnia that is due to a mismatch between the sleep–wake schedule required by a person's environment and his or her circadian sleep–wake pattern.

B. The sleep disturbance causes clinically significant distress or impairment in social, occupational, or other important areas of functioning.

C. The disturbance does not occur exclusively during the course of another Sleep Disorder or other mental disorder.

D. The disturbance is not due to the direct physiological effects of a substance (e.g., a drug of abuse, a medication) or a general medical condition.

Specify type:

Delayed Sleep Phase Type: a persistent pattern of late sleep onset and late awakening times, with an inability to fall asleep and awaken at a desired earlier time

Jet Lag Type: sleepiness and alertness that occur at an inappropriate time of day relative to local time, occurring after repeated travel across more than one time zone

Shift Work Type: insomnia during the major sleep period or excessive sleepiness during the major awake period associated with night shift work or frequently changing shift work

Unspecified Type

in those individuals suspected of having true DSPS. This treatment is the easiest to implement and to adhere to, and some cases do resolve. If the implementation of good sleep hygiene is ineffective, several other treatments are available:

• Bright-white light exposure immediately after awakening (sunlight or light from a bright light box at 10,000 lux for 30–45 minutes) will advance sleep onset effectively in many patients and may successfully treat DSPS. Periodic morning bright light exposure may also help to keep circadian rhythms synchronized (Terman et al. 1995).

- Melatonin, 0.5–5.0 mg in the evening for a few days, may help to advance circadian rhythms in DSPS (Kayumov et al. 2001) (but see cautions in Chapter 7).
- Chronotherapy, formerly the treatment of choice for DSPS, consists of placing the patient on a 27-hour day and progressively phase-delaying the sleep cycle about 3 hours each sleep–wake period, until sleep-onset time has been moved essentially around the clock to the time the patient considers the appropriate bedtime. The primary disadvantage of this treatment method is the disturbance in daily schedule required to complete the phase delay.

Up to 50% of patients with severe DSPS may not respond to conventional treatment (Regestein and Monk 1995). These patients might best be referred to a sleep disorders center.

Advanced Sleep Phase Syndrome

Advanced sleep phase syndrome is less common than DSPS. The typical patient complains of falling asleep at 8:00 P.M. or earlier and awakening between 3:00 and 5:00 A.M. The origin of this syndrome is not yet clear, but phase advance of body temperature and melatonin rhythms is suspected. The differential diagnosis includes 1) affective disorders, which are often associated with an apparent advance in aspects of sleep rhythms, and 2) a habitual pattern of early bedtime to avoid evening social interactions or responsibilities. Some evidence suggests that elderly persons may have an age-related physiological advance in the circadian sleep cycle (Czeisler et al. 1992).

Treatment

- Bright light therapy at 10,000 lux for 30–45 minutes in the evening (between 7:00 and 9:00 P.M.) should be used for advanced sleep phase syndrome.
- A nonsedating antidepressant, such as desipramine or a serotonin reuptake inhibitor, should be considered if significant depression is evident. The administration of this medication can

be coupled with a suggestion that the patient attempt to delay evening bedtime very slowly (i.e., by 15 minutes every few days).

- Chronotherapy, with the patient going to bed 3 hours earlier each night until the sleep cycle is phase-advanced back to a normal bedtime, has been reported to be effective in case reports.

Non-24-Hour Sleep–Wake Cycle

Some individuals (most of them blind persons) who cannot respond to light as a rhythm entrainer maintain a 25-hour circadian rhythm, which significantly interferes with adaptation to a conventional life. Occasionally, even longer periods (up to 30–50 hours) develop. Mentally retarded children are also at risk of developing non-24-hour circadian rhythms.

Differential diagnosis. Frequent stimulant abuse would appear to be the most frequent mimic of non-24-hour sleep–wake syndrome. The clinician must obtain an adequate drug history and instruct the patient to graph very carefully his or her periodicity of sleeping and waking. Lengthened but severely erratic sleep periods can be an aspect of a schizoid avoidance of social contact, as well as a symptom of sporadic hypnotic and alcohol abuse.

Treatment. Early-morning bright-white light exposure at 10,000 lux for 30–45 minutes should be tried in individuals with a non-24-hour sleep–wake cycle. If they do not respond to light, melatonin (0.5–1.0 mg at bedtime) can be added to the treatment regimen. Melatonin has been shown to be effective in entraining the circadian system in blind persons (Sack et al. 2000). Any evidence of drug abuse, personality disorder, or affective disorder should be treated appropriately.

Irregular Sleep–Wake Cycle

Normal circadian function can be severely impaired in a number of illnesses and conditions, including severe dementia, head injury, recovery from coma, recovery from drug and alcohol intoxication, severe depression, and persistent dependence on central nervous system (CNS) stimulants, CNS depressants, or hypnotics. Some mentally retarded or otherwise brain-damaged persons may have an irregular sleep–wake cycle.

Treatment.   The underlying condition should be appropriately treated first, and then regularity of the sleep–wake cycle should be reinforced with normal daytime activity, regular exercise, regular meals, and good sleep hygiene. Morning bright-white light treatment and melatonin, 0.5–1.0 mg at bedtime, would perhaps merit a trial. This syndrome may be quite resistant to treatment.

Shift Work Sleep Disorder

Presenting complaints

- Chronic fatigue, drowsiness, and impaired work performance
- Difficulty initiating sleep
- Decreased duration and poor quality of sleep
- Complaints of job stress, depression, emotional problems, and family life disruption
- Somatic complaints, especially those related to the gastrointestinal system (e.g., gastritis and constipation)
- Increased use of alcohol, tranquilizers, or sleeping pills to decrease stress and increase sleep time
- Excessive smoking and caffeine consumption to aid alertness

Clinical presentation.   The shift worker's most common complaints are difficulty initiating and maintaining sleep and poor sleep quality. These people may have chronic fatigue, be drowsy, and doze off at work in association with the disrupted sleep. They have an increased number of accidents and attention-related mistakes. Shift workers are also reported to have a higher incidence of chronic depression, emotional problems, family life dysfunction, excessive drug (including nicotine) and alcohol use, ulcers, and myocardial infarction than the general population.

Whereas some shift workers will seek help from employers or physicians, others have problems that come to light only after on-the-job accidents, falling asleep at work, detection of drug or alcohol use, development of medical complaints, or quitting to avoid shift work (Scott 2000). Shift workers' sleep symptoms have been termed *shift work sleep disorder* (or shift work maladaptation syndrome).

Incidence.   In 1991, it was estimated that approximately 20% of workers in the United States were working on nonstandard schedules ("Biological Rhythms" 1991), a percentage that is continually increasing as we move toward a 24/7 society. Of those working during the night shift, 75% are estimated to experience sleepiness every night, and 20% actually fall asleep periodically during their shifts (Akerstedt 1992). Alertness is most difficult to maintain at about the time of the core body temperature nadir. Epidemiological studies have suggested that about 25% of shift workers (or 5% of the American workforce) may have some aspect of a shift work maladaptation syndrome (Gordon et al. 1986).

Etiology and pathophysiology.   Shift work sleep disorder has been postulated to be caused by either disturbances in regulation of circadian rhythms, with internal desynchrony secondary to work shift time changes, or loss of sleep—or possibly both. Another major and related factor in the etiology of shift work sleep disorders is the disruption of family life by frequent absence, tiredness, depression, and the need to sleep during daytime hours.

A sudden work shift change of 8 hours causes the sleep–wake schedule to be suddenly out of synchronization with other circadian biorhythms. When the circadian physiology is desynchronized, sleep can be difficult to initiate, less restful when obtained, and more often interrupted and shortened in length. Being forced to function out of synchrony appears to "flatten" circadian biorhythms, and body temperature has less variation throughout the day. This flattening may contribute to a chronic inability to sustain normal sleep.

Investigators have also postulated that the sleep loss itself, with symptoms of sleep deprivation, and perhaps the means used to combat it (e.g., alcohol, sedatives) and reinforce alertness (e.g., stimulants, cigarettes, food) contribute to shift workers' symptoms.

Laboratory findings.   A PSG would typically show increased sleep latency, numerous arousals during sleep, and early awakening, as well as sleep efficiency below 85%. However, a PSG is usually not needed unless the clinician suspects an additional primary sleep disorder.

Differential diagnosis.   Because of the high incidence of emotional problems within the shift worker group, the therapist should evaluate the patient for affective and anxiety disorders that may require psychotherapy or medication and should take a careful medical and sleep history. A history of returning to a normal sleep pattern during vacations or time off rotation can help with diagnosis.

The clinician should examine the patient carefully for evidence of alcoholism or drug dependence, insomnia due to poor sleep hygiene such as excessive caffeine and cigarette use, or use of alcohol as a regular sedative. Many shift workers aggravate their conditions with poor sleep hygiene, which complicates diagnosis and treatment.

Treatment.   The body's ability to adapt to shift changes is in part a function of the direction of the shift, which determines whether a phase delay (easier to adapt to) or a phase advance (more difficult to adapt to) is required. A person needs about 3 days to adapt to an 8-hour shift change that allows sleep time to shift 8 hours later (phase delay). If the sleep time has to shift 8 hours earlier (phase advance), the person may require 6–7 days to adapt. Workers who have no regular shifts but are constantly on call may never have a chance to develop adequate synchrony.

Two general approaches to treatment include 1) treatment of the patient and 2) attempts to encourage the workplace to adapt to workers' needs.

Treatment recommendations for shift workers include the following:

- Attempt to maintain a regular sleep and meal schedule whenever possible.
- Take naps to limit sleep loss.
- Practice good sleep hygiene, including reducing alcohol and caffeine consumption. If sleep is necessary during daylight hours, ensure adequate darkness and screen noise and interruptions as much as possible.
- Pay attention to the light environment. Bright light during the first portion of the shift and protection from bright light after work and before sleep may be beneficial (Eastman et al. 1994, 1995).
- Take short-half-life hypnotics to help initiate sleep. However, hypnotics should be used primarily by those who only occasionally work shifts; hypnotic use on a chronic basis by long-term shift workers cannot be encouraged.

Recommendations for organizations that wish to adapt to workers' needs include the following:

- Allow workers to change shifts in a phase-delayed direction (i.e., night shift to day shift), which has been shown to result in improved worker satisfaction, productivity, and health (Czeisler et al. 1982).
- Encourage short naps, if appropriate, as a way to aid in maintaining alertness during long work stints.
- Avoid excessively long shifts whenever possible.
- Provide high-intensity lighting in the workplace, especially during the first part of the shift. Such lighting has been shown to improve alertness, efficiency, and worker satisfaction (Eastman et al. 1995).
- Institute a work-scheduling system such as the "European twos," which seems to be favored by workers over other longer-period work shift schedules (e.g., 1 week on each shift). In this system,

workers spend 2 days on each shift consecutively and then have 3 days off. Although circadian rhythms are maximally disrupted during the 2 days on night shift, workers can quickly return to their typical routine, and some claim to get more sleep with this system.

Jet Lag

Jet lag is a travel-induced circadian rhythm desynchronization in which sleep–wake and other circadian physiological rhythms are suddenly out of synchrony with the new 24-hour light–dark cycle. The body can adapt easily to a time change of about an hour a day; thus, no jet lag–like condition existed in times of slower travel. As travel speed increases and as time zones are crossed more rapidly, jet lag becomes a problem.

Symptoms of jet lag include difficulty sleeping at the new sleep time, daytime sleepiness and fatigue, and impaired performance during the new daylight hours. The body's 24-hour rhythms, such as those for serum cortisol and body temperature, remain on the old time and shift slowly to the new time, requiring about 1 day to adapt for each hour of time change. Jet lag symptoms are usually more pronounced for travel from west to east (which entails a phase advance) and less pronounced for travel from east to west (which entails a phase delay). Thus, travelers flying from the United States to Europe typically have more difficulty than those flying from Europe to the United States.

Treatment.   Treatment of jet lag includes both behavioral and pharmacological components. It is helpful to lead the time change by beginning to shift sleep and activity patterns ahead of time. In any case, it is best to change to the new rest–activity schedule immediately on arrival, sleeping at the new sleep time, eating at the new mealtimes, and working at the new work time.

Additional treatment may include the following measures:

• Take a short-acting hypnotic, such as zolpidem (5 mg at bedtime), for the first few nights to protect sleep at the new nighttime hours.

- Use appropriately timed exposure to bright light to speed adjustment to the new time zone (Czeisler et al. 1986). Decisions about when to get bright light (e.g., by being outdoors in sunlight) or when to avoid bright light (e.g., by staying indoors or wearing dark glasses) are based on the proposed phase-response curve (PRC) for bright light (see Chapter 2, Figure 2–9). Keeping in mind that the PRC transition point (point x) occurs near the time of core body temperature minimum (which usually occurs at about 4:00 to 5:00 A.M. in the *starting time zone*), one can plan periods of bright light exposure in the new time zone that either phase-delay or phase-advance the underlying circadian rhythm and thus change the time of sleep. For example, light exposure in area B of the PRC (occurring after the transition point) will cause a phase advance, which is helpful in west to east travel (see example of New York City to Paris, Figure 3–2). Light exposure in area A of the PRC (occurring before the transition point) will cause a phase delay, which is especially helpful in east to west travel (see example of Los Angeles to Hong Kong, Figure 3–2).
- Take a bedtime dose of melatonin (0.5–1.0 mg) for several days, which may help to reentrain the circadian system more rapidly.

■ PERIODIC LIMB MOVEMENT DISORDER AND RESTLESS LEGS SYNDROME

Presenting Complaints of Periodic Limb Movement Disorder

- Patient usually complains primarily of chronic insomnia, often with frequent awakenings or excessive daytime sleepiness.
- Patient may complain of leg jerking.
- Bed partner complains that patient kicks during sleep.
- Bedclothes are frequently in disarray in the morning.
- Patient may have associated restless legs symptoms.
- Patient's complaints can be aggravated by antidepressants.

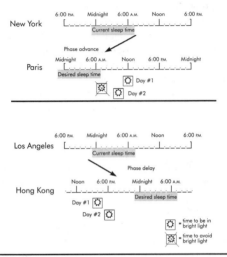

FIGURE 3–2. **Examples of how to use bright light to reentrain circadian system in west to east (phase advance) and east to west (phase delay) travel.**

Presenting Complaints of Restless Legs Syndrome

- Uncomfortable "crawling" feelings, usually in the calf of the leg, begin when the patient lies down to sleep.
- Crawling feelings are relieved by movement (e.g., walking).

Clinical Presentation

PLMD and RLS are considered together because they frequently occur together and may share certain features. *Periodic limb movement disorder* eventually was established as the official name of the disorder, which was originally called nocturnal myoclonus.

Patients with PLMD typically display periodic (every 20–40 seconds) stereotypic contractions of the tibialis anterior with muscle dorsiflexion of the ankle and toes, resulting in a leg jerk or a

slight kick, frequently accompanied by a short electroencephalographic arousal. The bed partner may complain that the patient is
very restless or that he or she kicks for prolonged periods during the
night. The patient usually is not aware of the leg jerks but is aware
only of the sense of being awake or waking frequently. Periodic
limb movements may also occur when the patient naps in a chair
during the day. PLMD may present as EDS, especially if nocturnal
sleep is severely fragmented by the leg jerks. The ICSD diagnostic
criteria for PLMD (780.52–4) are as follows:

A. The patient has a complaint of insomnia or excessive sleepi-
    ness. The patient occasionally will be asymptomatic, and the
    movements are noticed by an observer.
B. Repetitive highly stereotyped limb muscle movements are
    present; in the leg, these movements are characterized by exten-
    sion of the big toe in combination with partial flexion of the an-
    kle, knee, and sometimes hip.
C. Polysomnographic monitoring demonstrates:
    1. Repetitive episodes of muscle contraction (0.5–5 seconds
        in duration) separated by an interval of typically 20–40 sec-
        onds.
    2. Arousal or awakenings may be associated with the move-
        ments.
D. The patient has no evidence of a medical or mental disorder that
    can account for the primary complaint.
E. Other sleep disorders (e.g., obstructive sleep apnea syndrome)
    may be present but do not account for the movements.

Minimal criteria: A+B

  RLS is a dysesthesia characterized by uncomfortable "creepy-
crawly" sensations and/or prickly feelings in the calves of the legs
that occur when the patient lies down to rest or sleep and that can
be alleviated only by getting up and "walking them out." Thus RLS
may not be a true sleep disorder, because the symptoms appear during wakefulness, but it certainly does interfere with sleep, and the

patient frequently presents with a complaint of sleep-onset insomnia. The patient may have difficulty expressing the nature of the uncomfortable feelings in his or her legs and, at times, may describe the feeling in somewhat strange terms, such as *worms crawling*.

The ICSD diagnostic criteria for RLS (780.52–5) are as follows:

A. The patient has a complaint of an unpleasant sensation in the legs at night or difficulty in initiating sleep.
B. Disagreeable sensations of "creeping" inside the calves are present and are often associated with general aches and pains in the legs.
C. The discomfort is relieved by movement of the limbs.
D. Polysomnographic monitoring demonstrates limb movements at sleep onset.
E. There is no evidence of any medical or mental disorders that account for the movements.
F. Other sleep disorders may be present but do not account for the symptom.

Minimal criteria: A+B+C

Incidence

Coleman et al. (1982) analyzed 5,000 patient records from 11 sleep disorders centers and found that of the patients with insomnia, PLMD or RLS was the cause in 12%. RLS has variously been estimated to be related to up to 10% of the cases of chronic insomnia, especially in older patients with medical disorders, in whom the syndrome is more common. Normally sleeping subjects may experience periodic limb movements in sleep but may not complain of insomnia and, thus, have no disorder. The incidence of PLMD is higher in males and increases with age, with some studies reporting that up to 44% of subjects age 65 or older have periodic limb movements in sleep (PLMS) indices (number of limb jerks per hour of sleep) of 5 or greater (Ancoli-Israel et al. 1985). The incidence of PLMD is also higher in patients with narcolepsy or sleep apnea. Unpublished findings from our laboratory suggest that PLMD may be relatively common even in patients with chronic insomnia complaints who have been prescreened (by history only) for PLMD.

Etiology and Pathophysiology

In some cases, PLMD and RLS are apparently transmitted as an autosomal-dominant trait, with onset in the second decade and lifelong persistence. Both syndromes have been associated with various medical disorders, including peripheral neuropathies, anemia, uremia, and chronic pulmonary disease. RLS per se has been linked to vitamin and mineral deficiencies (low iron stores), uremia, and malignancy and has been estimated to occur in up to 30% of patients with rheumatoid arthritis (Reynolds et al. 1986). A familial syndrome of nocturnal painful cramping and leg jerking has been described as well (Jacobson et al. 1986). It can also run in families and appear in pregnancy. Syndromes similar to PLMD and RLS accompany Huntington's chorea and amyotrophic lateral sclerosis. PLMD may also be associated with a fibrositis syndrome termed *rheumatic pain modulation disorder,* with an accompanying nonrestorative alpha-delta-like sleep pattern. This disorder has a higher incidence in women than in men.

The pathophysiology of PLMD is unclear. The possible involvement of the dopamine system has been suggested by several studies, and researchers have observed that dopamine agonists are useful in treatment and that dopamine antagonists worsen the syndrome. Patients with RLS have low iron brain stores and increased brain transferrin concentrations, which suggests that the low iron levels in the brain may modulate RLS, even in the face of normal serum iron levels.

PLMS, with dorsiflexion of the ankle and toes, and sometimes fanning, is similar to the Babinski reflex. These movements are sometimes accompanied by changes in autonomic activity and electroencephalograms (EEGs), which suggest an origin similar to, if not the same as, that of the Babinski reflex. The Babinski reflex elicited during wakefulness is indicative of pyramidal tract disease, but it can normally be elicited during non-REM sleep, because inhibitory suprasegmental influences are suppressed during these sleep stages. Some evidence exists for increased segmental excitability of brain stem and spinal reflexes in patients with PLMD, which would implicate a mechanism at the pontine (or more rostral) level (Wechsler et al. 1986).

Laboratory Findings

For a movement to be scored as a periodic limb movement, the tibialis anterior electromyogram (EMG) should show bursts of activity of at least 0.5 seconds, but not more than 5.0 seconds, in duration. At least two such electromyographic bursts must occur within a 4- to 90-second interval (usually 20–40 seconds) for a leg jerk to be counted. The total number of leg jerks occurring during sleep is divided by the number of hours of sleep to provide a myoclonic index or PLMS index. Myoclonic activity typically occurs in bouts during the night. Thus, for example, a bout of 30–60 or more periodic limb movements may be followed by fairly normal sleep for 1 hour or more, only to be followed by another bout of periodic limb movements. The number of periodic limb movements can vary significantly from night to night, which complicates assessment by sleep laboratory studies. In most patients with RLS, PLMS is also seen on a PSG (80%–87%), but not all patients with PLMD complain of RLS.

The PLMS index must be interpreted in the context of other clinical and polysomnographic findings. Periodic limb movements accompanied by evidence of arousal (alpha activity in the EEG, increase in chin muscle activity in the EMG) are of more concern than episodes showing no arousal; polysomnographic records should be scored and interpreted accordingly, with leg jerks associated with arousals separated from those not associated with arousals. It is difficult to define an abnormal PLMS index (or associated arousal index). The polysomnographic finding must be viewed with the entire clinical scenario in mind before treatment is instituted. Most laboratories use a cutoff of five leg jerks per hour as the upper limit of normal. Patients with severe disease can have more than 100 leg jerks per hour. Examples of periodic limb movements without and with arousal are illustrated in Figures 3–3 and 3–4, respectively.

Differential Diagnosis

RLS is diagnosed by the history. PLMD can also be suggested by the history, but a PSG is required for definitive diagnosis. Patients treated for chronic insomnia, without benefit of a PSG, may have undiagnosed PLMD. Therefore, this diagnosis should be suspected in patients not responding to other insomnia treatments, especially if they have a pattern of sleep-maintenance insomnia.

Specific conditions to consider in the differential diagnosis of PLMD include

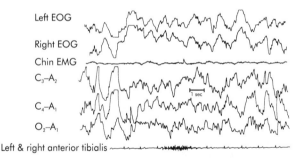

FIGURE 3–3. **Polysomnogram showing periodic limb movement not accompanied by arousal.**

Leg jerk indicated by electromyographic burst in left and right leg (combined) tibialis anterior electromyogram (EMG) (bottom channel). Ongoing Stage III sleep is not disrupted (no arousal).

A_1=left ear; A_2=right ear; C_3=left high central electroencephalogram (EEG); C_4=right high central EEG; EOG=electro-oculogram; O_2=right occipital EEG.

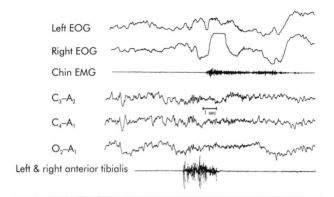

FIGURE 3–4. **Polysomnogram showing periodic limb movement accompanied by arousal.**

Leg jerk in tibialis anterior electromyogram (EMG) (bottom channel) is followed by electroencephalographic arousal, with increased chin muscle activity (EMG) and eye movement.

A_1=left ear; A_2=right ear; C_3=left high central electroencephalogram (EEG); C_4=right high central EEG; EOG=electro-oculogram; O_2=right occipital EEG.

- *Hypnic jerks,* which are sudden body jerks that often occur at sleep onset and are frequently accompanied by imagery such as missing a step. These sleep-onset phenomena, also called *sleep starts,* are similar to a startle reaction and are considered to be normal phenomena.

- *Nocturnal leg cramps in the calves and in the muscles of the sole of the foot,* "charley horses," which are usually relieved by stretching. Occasionally, severe nocturnal cramps also may respond to quinine, a low dose of codeine, diphenhydramine, or verapamil at bedtime. There may be familial versions of this disorder that, if frequent, may respond to clonazepam, 0.25 mg at bedtime.

- *Peripheral vascular insufficiency,* which may have associated nocturnal leg cramps. An evaluation for arteriosclerotic disease may be indicated.

- *Peripheral neuropathy,* with associated burning pain and discomfort.
- *Other myoclonic-like activities associated with CNS degenerative conditions,* which should be apparent on physical examination.
- *Painful legs and moving toes syndrome,* which is a rare syndrome that includes neuropathic pain in the feet and spontaneous movement of the toes (Spillane et al. 1971).
- *Epileptic myoclonus,* which is usually associated with electroencephalographic abnormalities.
- *Nocturnal cataclysms* (Myers et al. 1986), which are frightening nocturnal episodes that have reportedly accompanied clomipramine use. These episodes have been relieved by clonazepam.
- *Episodic fragmentary myoclonus,* which is a rare disorder seen predominantly in males and is characterized by brief (<150 milliseconds), random, multifocal, asynchronous muscle jerks occurring predominantly during non-REM sleep, with a clinical complaint of either insomnia or EDS (Broughton et al. 1985).

Arthritic or muscular pain, neuroleptic-induced akathisia, and opiate withdrawal are other differential concerns to consider.

Perhaps the major problem in clinical assessment of PLMD is determining to what degree the leg movements contribute to the overall sleep complaint. Nocturnal myoclonus as an isolated finding in the absence of sleep complaints is called *essential nocturnal myoclonus.* When insomnia or hypersomnia is the complaint, however, the clinician must use his or her clinical skills to estimate to what extent leg movements contribute to the sleep complaint and whether other causes of the sleep complaint may coexist, such as a psychophysiological or learned insomnia or a concurrent psychiatric disorder. Treatment for more than one disorder may be necessary.

Treatment

The drugs most commonly used in first-line treatment for RLS and PLMD are dopaminergic agents (Hering et al. 1999). The drug that has been primarily studied is levodopa, most commonly in combination with carbidopa or benserazide. Newer-generation dopaminergic drugs such as pergolide, pramipexole, and ropinirole have been quite popular, in part because of a study showing pergolide to be superior to levodopa. These agents reduce periodic limb movements, decrease leg restlessness, and improve sleep quality. Typical starting doses for these agents and others are listed in Table 3–4. Opioids have been shown to be effective in reducing leg jerking movements as well as eliminating the sensation of limb restlessness. Oxycodone seems to be most commonly used and may be more effective than other drugs; typical dosage is 10–15 mg/day. One must be quite cautious with patients who request opiate treatment for subjectively restless legs. Still, most experience shows that RLS patients seldom need to increase opiate doses after many years. Propoxyphene is beneficial, but it is not as effective as oxycodone or dopaminergic agents. Benzodiazepines have frequently been used for RLS and PLMD. Clonazepam was introduced with the idea that a "myoclonic" event necessitates use of an anticonvulsant. Benzodiazepines tend to work by offering sedation to inhibit awakenings secondary to frequent movements; sleep quality therefore improves.

The anticonvulsants carbamazepine and gabapentin as well as the α-adrenergic blocker clonidine have all been shown to offer relief for patients with RLS. Folic acid has also been effective for RLS in some patients.

In a small experimental study, six of eight patients with RLS responded quite well to intravenous administration of iron (Earley et al. 2001). This finding supports the hypothesis that decreased brain iron stores may be a cause of RLS. Further studies will clarify the role of intravenous iron therapy as a first-line treatment for RLS or PLMD.

Many individuals taking levodopa develop a rebound of their symptoms later in the night or even the next day. This rebound effect, also termed *augmentation,* can usually be managed by both behavioral strategies (encouraging walking and other physical activity) and medication-timing strategies (Allen and Earley 1996). This effect may also, however, necessitate a change in medication to opioids.

TABLE 3–4. **Typical starting doses of drugs used for PLMD and RLS**

Drug	Starting dose (mg)	Time of administration
Carbidopa/Levodopa	25/100 to 50/200	Bedtime or when symptoms occur
Controlled-release carbidopa/levodopa	25/100 to 50/200	Bedtime or when symptoms occur
Oxycodone	5–15	Bedtime
Codeine	10–60	Bedtime
Bromocriptine	2.5–5	Bedtime
Triazolam	0.125–0.25	Bedtime
Temazepam	15–30	Bedtime
Clonazepam	0.5–1.5	Bedtime
Baclofen	20–40	Bedtime
Pergolide	0.05	Bedtime or when symptoms occur
Pramipexole	0.125	Bedtime
Ropinirole	0.25	Bedtime
Gabapentin	100–300	Bedtime

Note. Lowest doses are initiated with titration on the basis of clinical response. PLMD=periodic limb movement disorder; RLS=restless legs syndrome.

Combining an agent to decrease RLS (e.g., levodopa) with an agent to improve sleep continuity (e.g., a hypnotic) is sometimes successful. Clinicians are advised also to refer to the recently published AASM practice parameters for treatment of RLS and PLMD (Chesson et al. 1999b).

Other treatment strategies.   The treatment of PLMD coexisting with other disorders such as sleep-related breathing disorders, narcolepsy, or sleep complaints related to affective disorders is complicated by the fact that tricyclic antidepressants and selective serotonin reuptake inhibitors, often used in the treatment of these disorders, may substantially increase periodic limb movements. Lithium has also been reported to increase leg movements.

Biofeedback aimed at increasing skin temperature of the foot has been reported to diminish sleep complaints in PLMD patients who complain of cold feet. This option, if available, might be considered for selected patients (Ancoli-Israel et al. 1986).

The multiplicity of proposed treatments suggests that the optimum treatment strategy might begin with administration of the most innocuous agent and proceed to use of more active compounds only if required. The clinician must observe for, and alert patients to, possible side effects and drug complications.

■ SLEEP APNEA INSOMNIA

Presenting Complaints

- Insomnia, with sleep disruption and frequent awakenings
- Possible complaints of depression and/or decreased libido
- Occasional complaints of difficulty getting a breath, or gasping
- Occasional complaints of snoring

Clinical Presentation

Patients with frequent central apneas during sleep may present with a complaint of insomnia. Associated symptoms can include snoring, depression, and decreased libido. These patients usually do not have EDS or other manifestations typical of the obstructive apnea syndrome. Patients most often have no direct respiratory complaint, although occasionally they have a sense of momentary breathlessness, difficulty getting a breath, or gasping respiration (not true shortness of breath). The bed partner will frequently give a history of repeated short pauses in the patient's respiration during sleep.

Incidence

Studies of the presence of significant central apnea in adult insomniac populations have found incidences ranging from 1% to 12%; our experience is compatible with the lower end of this range.

Although central apnea is probably among the rarer causes of chronic insomnia in younger patients, its incidence increases with advancing age, as does the incidence of mixed and obstructive apneas (Ancoli-Israel et al. 1987).

Central apneas that occur alone are relatively uncommon; more frequently, they occur in combination with obstructive apneas or as antecedents to obstructive events, in which case they are termed *mixed apneas.*

The incidence of central apnea (or periodic breathing) increases at higher elevations, and sleep-related respiratory disturbances may account for many of the sleep complaints experienced by most individuals during the first several nights at high altitude (e.g., while camping, mountain climbing, or on a skiing vacation).

Etiology and Pathophysiology

Central apneas occur when the respiratory efforts of the diaphragm and intercostal muscles cease, and breathing is momentarily interrupted. The apneas are usually terminated by a brief arousal, thus producing sleep fragmentation, the subjective sense of not sleeping, and the complaint of insomnia. These apneas, as seen on an EEG, frequently occur at the transition point between wakefulness and Stage I sleep.

Respiration during sleep is closely related to the activity of chemoreceptors, including the carotid body for hypoxia and medullary chemosensors for hypercapnia. Individuals with abnormally functioning chemosensors (e.g., patients with Ondine's curse) may hypoventilate during the day and have respiratory abnormalities, including both central and obstructive apneas, during sleep. Hypoxia may increase breathing rate during sleep, and pCO_2 is thought to be a major factor in the maintenance of respiratory regularity during sleep. If pCO_2 levels decrease for whatever reason (e.g., hyperventilation secondary to hypoxia at high altitude), irregular or periodic breathing and, possibly, central apnea ensue. The sleep state itself appears to be associated with a depression in both hypoxic and hypercapnic ventilatory drives, which may account for the association between sleep–wake transitions and central apneas. The presence of central apnea does not necessarily imply a disorder of the chemosensors, because patients with substantial apnea may have normally functioning chemosensors (White 1985).

The hemodynamic consequences of central apneas are not as profound as those of obstructive or mixed apneas. Oxygen desaturation is relatively slight, and relatively small increases in pulmonary artery pressure and systemic pressure have been described as accompanying central apneas.

Central apneas may accompany several medical disorders, including congestive heart failure, diabetes mellitus, nasal obstruction (from either anatomical abnormalities or nasal congestion due to a common cold), and several neurological disorders, among them familial dysautonomia, Shy-Drager syndrome, encephalitis, and brain stem tumors or infarctions.

Laboratory Findings

Central apneas are defined as loss of both respiratory effort and flow for a period of at least 10 seconds (see Chapter 4, Figure 4–4). Most central apneas tend to be short (<20 seconds) and have minimal hemodynamic consequences. A nocturnal PSG with a central apnea index of more than 5 in a patient complaining of chronic insomnia should be considered evidence that the apneas could be contributing to the insomnia complaint. Apnea indices are sometimes considerably greater than 5, with several hundred apneas occurring during the night. In such cases, the relation of the apnea to the insomnia complaint is clearer, and the clinician is more comfortable attributing the insomnia to the apnea.

Differential Diagnosis

Insomnia based on central apnea is essentially a sleep laboratory diagnosis. The therapist's index of suspicion is heightened when patients complain of a sense of difficulty getting their breath or of breathlessness on waking (Table 3–5). Snoring, or a bed partner's complaint that the patient breathes irregularly or stops breathing, should also increase the index of suspicion. Once central sleep apnea is diagnosed on the basis of a PSG, the clinician should evaluate the patient for treatable causes such as congestive heart failure, nasal obstruction, and other less common causes (listed earlier). The more common sleep-related breathing disorders associated with EDS are discussed in Chapter 4.

More common perhaps is the situation in which a patient with other causes of insomnia has a minimally increased number of central apneas. In this situation, contributing factors such as anxiety, psychological factors, stress, and evidence of a psychophysiological insomnia come into play. In such cases, it is important not to overtreat the apnea or to place too much emphasis initially on central apnea as the major cause of the insomnia. Rather, the treatment strategy should emphasize efforts aimed at the other possible causative factors, as appropriate.

Treatment

The treatment of central sleep apnea is not entirely satisfactory. If central apneas occur along with obstructive events, treatment is directed at the obstructive event, and the central apneas often resolve as well. If medical problems (e.g., congestive heart failure or nasal obstruction) are identifiable, then they should be treated first.

TABLE 3–5. **DSM-IV-TR diagnostic criteria for breathing-related sleep disorder**

A. Sleep disruption, leading to excessive sleepiness or insomnia, that is judged to be due to a sleep-related breathing condition (e.g., obstructive or central sleep apnea syndrome or central alveolar hypoventilation syndrome).

B. The disturbance is not better accounted for by another mental disorder and is not due to the direct physiological effects of a substance (e.g., a drug of abuse, a medication) or another general medical condition (other than a breathing-related disorder).

Coding note: Also code sleep-related breathing disorder on Axis III.

In a number of studies, supplemental oxygen (1–2 L/minute via a nasal cannula) proved to be helpful, even in patients with minimal desaturations during the diagnostic study. Nasal continuous positive airway pressure has also been shown to be effective in some patients with central sleep apnea, as well as in others with Cheyne-Stokes respiration, which is associated with congestive heart failure. The mechanism of action may involve the increase of pCO_2 levels above the apneic threshold during sleep.

In short-term trials, acetazolamide (a carbonic anhydrase inhibitor) 125–250 mg two to three times daily has shown some success in treating central sleep apnea. It has also proven helpful in treating central sleep apnea with ascent to altitude. Some patients have been reported to develop obstructive apnea while taking acetazolamide; thus, follow-up sleep studies are prudent in certain cases.

Some individuals have central apnea consistently before and after arousals. If there is no significant oxygen desaturation, a trial of a hypnotic agent (e.g., zolpidem, 5–10 mg) may help to decrease the number of arousals and subsequent apneas. It may be advisable to repeat a PSG while the patient is taking hypnotic drugs, to verify that hypoxia is not worsening. In some cases, nocturnal ventilation via a tracheostomy or nasal mask may be necessary.

■ PRIMARY INSOMNIA

Although there are several more unusual causes of chronic insomnia, it is generally safe to assume that once the foregoing categories (medical- or psychiatric-related insomnia, substance abuse–related insomnia, circadian rhythm–based sleep disorder, PLMD, and central apnea) have been systematically excluded, we are in all probability left with a possible primary insomnia diagnosis (DSM-IV-TR 307.42). In the past, the condition of such patients tended to be subsumed under the terms *psychophysiological, learned,* or *conditioned insomnia.* Another syndrome related to primary insomnia consists of individuals who complain of insomnia but who, when studied in the sleep laboratory, demonstrate normal sleep. This is termed *sleep state misperception syndrome* and may actually represent different conditions and may benefit from separate consideration.

DSM-IV-TR diagnostic criteria for primary insomnia are presented in Table 3–6.

TABLE 3–6.	**DSM-IV-TR diagnostic criteria for primary insomnia**

A. The predominant complaint is difficulty initiating or maintaining sleep, or nonrestorative sleep, for at least 1 month.

B. The sleep disturbance (or associated daytime fatigue) causes clinically significant distress or impairment in social, occupational, or other important areas of functioning.

C. The sleep disturbance does not occur exclusively during the course of Narcolepsy, Breathing-Related Sleep Disorder, Circadian Rhythm Sleep Disorder, or a Parasomnia.

D. The disturbance does not occur exclusively during the course of another mental disorder (e.g., Major Depressive Disorder, Generalized Anxiety Disorder, a delirium).

E. The disturbance is not due to the direct physiological effects of a substance (e.g., a drug of abuse, a medication) or a general medical condition.

Clinical Presentation

Primary insomnia presents as a quite persistent disorder, often not previously responsive to treatment. The term *psychophysiological insomnia* or *conditioned insomnia* (sometimes *learned insomnia*) describes a condition in which patients (often those who have never been good sleepers) typically develop a chronic insomnia after a period of stress and continue to experience this insomnia even after the stress remits. Some patients may condition themselves not to sleep (see the section entitled "Etiology and Pathophysiology"); that is, they may "learn" the insomnia. More specifically, they learn a conditioned arousal to the normal sleep environment. Sleep complaints tend to be fixed over time, but they may covary with the degree of daytime stress. Such patients often tend to be tense or "wired" individuals; thus, there may be some overlap with primary insomnia. Sleep-onset insomnia does not always characterize this disorder. These patients can usually fall asleep rather easily, but then they may have several hours of wakefulness later in the night.

Incidence

Primary insomnia represents a relatively new diagnostic category, and thus accurate incidence and prevalence figures are not available. However, several studies have estimated that more than 20% of adults experience a bout of chronic insomnia at some time during their lives (Lugaresi et al. 1986), and a large proportion of those cases might be expected to fall into this diagnostic category.

Etiology and Pathophysiology

Patients with primary insomnia present with impaired sleep as well as the associated symptoms such as increased body temperature (Adam et al. 1986), heart rate (Monroe 1967), and possibly metabolic rate (Bonnet and Arand 1995). These symptoms all reflect a state of CNS hyperarousal in which case the insomnia complaint is likely one symptom of a more complex underlying disorder. Regestein and colleagues (1993) found that patients with primary insomnia had increased amplitudes of the auditory evoked potential component P1N1, which correlated with scores on a 26-item hyperarousal scale, and that they also had greater electroencephalographic activity across the frequency spectrum. Lamarche and Ogilvie (1997) found evidence, based on electroencephalographic patterns during the sleep-onset period, that individuals with primary or psychophysiological insomnia have high cortical arousal. This may contribute to their difficulty in discriminating wakefulness from sleep. Some evidence supports abnormalities of melatonin rhythms in primary insomnia (Hajak et al. 1995). One would assume (although confirmatory data do not yet exist) that a condition of chronic sleep deprivation with associated symptoms of insufficient sleep would be an additional complication of such a disorder.

Conditioned arousal (a term still sometimes used interchangeably with *psychophysiological insomnia*) characteristically begins when a susceptible individual experiences a stress-related transient insomnia and after several nights of poor sleep begins to fear going to bed because of the concerns that sleep will once again be difficult to initiate or maintain. This fear is associated with increased arousal, and soon a vicious cycle is established in which merely going into the bedroom to prepare for sleep results in a conditioned arousal response sufficient to interfere with sleep. The conditioned arousal can persist long after the stress that caused the initial transient insomnia has resolved. Often the conditioned arousal is limited to the individual's own bedroom and might not be transferred to other sleeping locations. Such patients may be able to sleep on the living room couch, for example, and they may not necessarily have difficulty napping during the day or sleeping while on vacation in a new environment. Conditioned insomnia appears to occur most often in individuals who have a history of "fragile sleep" (stressful events have been prone to interfere with their sleep), and such individuals may be prone to develop primary insomnia.

Life stress events appear to play a role in the development of chronic insomnia. Patients with chronic insomnia tend to have had a greater number of life stress events during the year that their insomnia began, particularly events related to loss and ill health (Healey et al. 1981). It is not clear whether these individuals, for whatever reason, are not as able as persons without insomnia to handle stressful life events.

Laboratory Findings

When studied in the sleep laboratory, most patients with primary insomnia will have a prolonged sleep latency (>30 minutes), frequent awakenings, a short TST (<6 hours), and low sleep efficiency (<85%), as well as a shift to lighter sleep stages on a PSG. Some patients will have a mild tachycardia (80–90 beats per minute) during slow-wave sleep, which suggests increased autonomic arousal. However, to date, no specific set of physiological findings is pathognomonic of primary insomnia. Subjects with psychophysiological insomnia may have a similar set of sleep abnormalities, suggesting an overlap with primary insomnia in those with a learned or conditioned component. They may also, however, have a relatively normal PSG, which suggests that a conditioned component (to their own sleep environment) is paramount and that a primary insomnia component may not be present.

Normal sleep on a PSG also raises the question of a possible sleep state misperception syndrome. Most often, however, a patient with a conditioned or learned insomnia who sleeps normally in the laboratory will comment that the sleep in the laboratory was an unusually good night of sleep, and the patient will be able to differentiate it from his or her usual nighttime insomnia. A patient with sleep state misperception syndrome, on the other hand, will still complain that the night spent in the sleep laboratory was illustrative of his or her usual poor sleep, even though it may have been objectively quite normal. In experimental laboratory studies, when these individuals are awakened from Stage III–IV sleep, they frequently report that they were, in fact, already awake; thus, they may not be accurately recognizing the sleep state (Mendelson 1993). Bonnet and Arand (1995) described evidence of increased metabolism in subjects with sleep state misperception syndrome, and the authors raised the possibility that this syndrome may represent either a milder version of or a natural precursor to a primary insomnia disorder.

There is no clear and agreed-on demarcation between a conditioned arousal insomnia and primary insomnia characterized by evidence of physiological hyperarousal. Both conditions were previously subsumed under the term *psychophysiological insomnia,* a term suggesting greater pathophysiological understanding than in fact exists. Indeed, it is likely that there is overlap, in that both conditions appear to be characterized by a state of hyperarousal. Treatment should focus on the hyperarousal, whose etiology may not always be apparent.

Differential Diagnosis

The clinician should first establish that the patient has a true insomnia (Table 3–6) and is not merely a typical short sleeper. Short sleepers, although not common, do exist and may get along fine on 4–5 hours of sleep a night. They do not complain of EDS or fatigue, and usually they have no sleep complaints. The family of a short sleeper, however, sees the patient up until midnight and then out of bed again at 4:00 A.M., assumes that he or she has a sleep problem, and convinces him or her to seek professional help. Short sleepers need no specific treatment, although an explanation is helpful for family members.

Similarly, the clinician should ascertain that a true insomnia is in fact present, rather than just a subjective sleep disturbance caused by poor sleep habits or an atypical or erratic sleep schedule. Shift workers, or people with very erratic sleep schedules for various reasons (e.g., computer hackers who like to work at night), frequently complain of poor sleep, which can be traced to their irregular sleep schedules. The shift work sleep disorder is a more chronic syndrome that includes prominent sleep complaints (see the section "Shift Work Sleep Disorder," earlier in this chapter).

The complaint of insomnia without objective findings, *sleep state misperception syndrome* (sometimes previously termed *pseudoinsomnia*), is encountered occasionally. Such individuals often present with a history compatible with psychophysiological insomnia; however, when their sleep is studied in the sleep laboratory, it is found to be normal, even in the face of their continued complaint of poor sleep. The insomnia complaint should be viewed seriously in these individuals, even though polysomnographic findings do not indicate disturbed sleep. Occasionally, the information that sleep, as characterized on the PSG, was found to be normal is helpful to such patients, but more typically a course of treatment as outlined for psychophysiological insomnia (see "Treatment") is indicated.

Primary insomnia as a cause of chronic insomnia should not be diagnosed until other causes have been excluded, including drug dependence, PLMD, central sleep apnea, psychiatric causes, poor sleep habits, and circadian rhythm disorders.

The diagnosis may be complicated when a sleep disturbance has multiple etiologies or is accompanied by poor sleep habits. The frequent addition of a learned or conditioned insomnia–type over-lay to other types of insomnia also must be considered.

Treatment

Treatment of primary insomnia, as well as of psychophysiological insomnia, includes both behavioral and pharmacological components. Behavioral components include sleep hygiene, self-control techniques, relaxation training, biofeedback, sleep restriction, and cognitive therapies. Practice parameters have recently been developed for the behavioral treatment of insomnia (Chesson et al. 1999a).

Behavioral Components

Sleep Hygiene.   Sleep hygiene should be emphasized in the treatment of any chronic insomnia, including psychophysiological insomnia. Good sleep hygiene, as summarized in Table 3–7, includes the following:

TABLE 3–7.   **Sleep hygiene**

Regular sleep time
Proper sleep environment
Wind-down time
Stimulus control
Avoidance of time in bed worrying
Avoidance of poorly timed alcohol and caffeine
Late-night high-tryptophan snack
Regular exercise but not within 3 hours of bedtime

- *Regular sleep time:* Establishing a regular sleep–wake schedule is very important, especially a regular time to awaken in the morning, with no more than a ±1-hour deviation from day to day, including weekends. Arousal time is perhaps the most important synchronizer of circadian rhythms. Awakening at 6:00 A.M. on weekdays to go to work and then sleeping until noon on weekends should be discouraged.

- *Proper sleep environment:* The bedroom should be cool, dark, and quiet. The clinician needs to inquire specifically about noise, because patients may habituate to a noisy sleep environment and may not remember the noise, even though it continues to disrupt their sleep patterns. Sleep interruptions should be minimized. Patients who have convinced themselves that they can sleep only with the radio or television on should be discouraged from this practice. Attention to the radio or television may prevent their minds from wandering or may keep them from beginning to worry about other matters, and thus positively affect sleep latency, but the continuing noise will be a disruptive factor during the night. Television and radios that automatically turn off may be useful.

- *Wind-down time:* Time to wind down before sleep is important. The clinician should advise patients to stop work at least 30 minutes before sleep-onset time and to change their activities to something different and nonstressful, such as reading or listening to music.

- *Stimulus control:* Patients should remove from the bedroom all stimuli that are not associated with sleep. The bedroom should be used for sleep and, of course, sexual activity (which is often conducive to sleep). Activities such as eating, drinking, arguing, discussing the day's problems, and paying bills should be done elsewhere, because their associated arousal may interfere with sleep onset.

- *Avoidance of time in bed worrying:* Patients should be encouraged not to remain in bed worrying about not being able to sleep or about activities that may be planned for the next day. If patients find themselves unable to sleep after 30 minutes, they should get up, read or complete a task, and then return to bed after they note the onset of sleepiness. Remaining in bed trying to fight wakefulness can further aggravate a conditioned arousal to the sleep setting.

- *Avoidance of poorly timed alcohol and caffeine:* Caffeine is quite disruptive of nocturnal sleep in many patients, and it may have a long half-life. Thus, caffeine consumption should be limited to the morning. A glass of wine or beer in the evening may help some individuals relax, but regularly having several drinks before bedtime for the express purpose of using the alcohol as a sedative should be discouraged. Alcohol in large doses can substantially disrupt and fragment sleep. Cigarette smoking may produce or aggravate insomnia in some patients.

- *Late-night high-tryptophan snack:* A bedtime snack such as a glass of milk, a cookie, a banana, or a similar high-tryptophan food may help promote sleep onset in some patients.
- *Regular exercise:* Exercising 20–30 minutes at least 3–4 days a week should be encouraged. Improved aerobic fitness has been shown experimentally to promote slow-wave sleep. Exercise should not occur within 3 hours of bedtime, however, because the autonomic arousal accompanying the exercise may delay sleep onset.

Self-Control Techniques.   Self-control techniques are important because many patients with chronic insomnia are considerably frustrated that they cannot control their sleep–wake patterns and feel out of control when they are unable to sleep at night. Such patients are more comfortable when they are in control of their lives in general, with respect to both daytime activity and sleep. This information usually can be elicited in an interview by direct questioning. For these patients, clinicians should consider—as part of a comprehensive insomnia treatment program—treatment strategies designed to enhance a sense of self-control. These treatment strategies may include supportive therapy aimed at dealing with control issues, autogenic training, relaxation tapes or training in progressive relaxation, or a recommendation that the patient participate in a meditation training program that fosters a sense of self-control.

Biofeedback.   Biofeedback treatment that directly teaches patients how to control autonomic function may be a useful therapeutic strategy (Hauri et al. 1983). Biofeedback may serve the dual function of enhancing a sense of self-control and reducing autonomic arousal. Although electromyographic and skin temperature biofeedback systems are perhaps the most commonly available forms, EEG theta biofeedback has been shown to be useful in tense, anxious patients with psychophysiological insomnia. EEG sensorimotor rhythm biofeedback has been found to be useful in patients with psychophysiological insomnia who are not particularly tense or anxious but who nonetheless have trouble sleeping. Sensorimotor rhythm biofeedback is at present rarely available, however. Some therapists believe that patients who are most likely to benefit from biofeedback include those who have demonstrated the ability to persevere and master difficult challenges (e.g., have achieved success in music as a child or in academic ventures).

Sleep Restriction. Patients with chronic insomnia (especially older patients) frequently spend greater and greater amounts of time in bed achieving less and less sleep; they may be in bed 10 hours or more and sleep only 6 hours. Sleep tends to spread out among the hours spent in bed, and this process further fragments nocturnal sleep. The principle of sleep restriction is to decrease substantially the time spent in bed so that sleep will consolidate to that time (Spielman et al. 1987). Restricting time available for sleep results in enhanced consolidation, which has important benefits in terms of improving actual and perceived sleep quality, as well as improving a subjective sense of self-control over sleep habits—an important consideration. The steps involved include the following:

1. Have the patient maintain a sleep diary for at least 5 nights. This diary should include the time to bed at night, the estimated time of sleep onset, the number and estimated time of awakenings during the night, the time of final awakening in the morning, and the time out of bed. From these 5-night sleep diary data, calculate the mean value for estimated TST and the percentage sleep efficiency: (TST/total time in bed) × 100.
2. Set the beginning total time in bed to equal the mean TST. For example, if the patient's estimate of his or her TST per night averaged over 5 nights is 5.5 hours, set the time in bed to no more than 5.5 hours, perhaps having the patient go to bed at 12:30

A.M. and get up again at 6:00 A.M. This restriction will result in increased daytime sleepiness the first several days, so the patient may need encouragement to continue with the program.

3. Instruct the patient to call in, usually to an answering machine, every morning while in the program and report his or her sleep data for the previous night, including time to bed, time of awakenings during sleep, time of final awakening, and time out of bed.

4. Calculate TST and sleep efficiency for each night. When mean sleep efficiency for 5 consecutive nights reaches 85% or better, increase time in bed by 15 minutes by allowing the patient to go to bed 15 minutes earlier. If mean sleep efficiency declines to less than 85%, decrease time in bed by 15 minutes (but not within the first 10 days of treatment). Naps outside the prescribed time in bed are not allowed.

5. Repeat the above procedure until the patient is maintaining a sleep efficiency of 85% or better and obtaining what he or she considers to be a subjectively adequate amount of nocturnal sleep.

Sleep restriction results in some unavoidable sleepiness at the beginning of the regimen, and not all patients can complete this treatment. However, those who do will have a substantial chance of improving their sleep efficiency.

Relaxation and Cognitive Therapy. Formal relaxation training and cognitive therapy have been shown to help with chronic insomnia, but both require considerable practitioner education and may not be practical in a primary care setting. Referral to an experienced psychologist may facilitate such treatment strategies.

Pharmacological Components

Pharmacological components of the insomnia treatment regimen might include a short-half-life nonbenzodiazepine hypnotic such as zolpidem (5–10 mg at bedtime). The ultra-short-acting agent zaleplon (10 mg) can be taken for middle-of-the-night awakenings, as long as 4 hours remain before rising. Zolpidem and zaleplon have the advantages of diminished tolerance, little evidence of rebound even after sustained use, and little impairment in memory or psychomotor function. Alternatively, the clinician may consider prescribing benzodiazepines such as triazolam (0.125 mg at bedtime), temazepam (15 mg at bedtime), or estazolam (1–2 mg at bedtime). Clinicians must remember that benzodiazepines produce tolerance, cause rebound symptoms if suddenly discontinued, and may adversely affect memory and psychomotor function. In the absence of other medical or psychiatric indications, it is preferable that the hypnotic not be used every night but rather two to three times per week as needed. Patients should be cautioned about not carrying out complex psychomotor tasks until the hypnotic action is concluded. As a guide, the U.S. Army will permit performance of aviation flight crew duties 12 hours after temazepam has been taken, 9 hours after triazolam has been taken, and 8 hours after zolpidem has been taken. Zaleplon ceases to impair function 4 hours after ingestion. The use of hypnotics is described further in Chapter 7.

In addition to the conventional hypnotic agents, sedative antidepressants such as certain tricyclics, trazodone, and mirtazapine often play an important role in the treatment of chronic insomnia. Tricyclics are frequently indicated for sleep problems related to affective disorders but are often useful in other insomnias as well (Ware 1983). In the experience of a number of clinicians (although no controlled double-blind studies have yet been done), a tricyclic can often be of benefit to a patient with chronic sleep-maintenance insomnia or early-morning awakening, especially if a degree of dysphoria or depressive affect seems to be present (often the case in many patients with chronic insomnia). Sedative tricyclics such as amitriptyline, nortriptyline, trimipramine, and doxepin, which are strongly antihistaminic, are often used. Special caution should be used in the case of patients who have increased risk factors such as cardiac conduction defects, glaucoma, or seizure disorders.

When tricyclic antidepressants are indicated, we often begin with nortriptyline (10–25 mg at bedtime) and increase the dose to 75 mg or more at bedtime; beneficial effects are often seen within several days. If the patient can tolerate the more sedating amitriptyline, beneficial sleep effects may be seen with the first dose.

Several advantages of tricyclics include their low abuse potential and their relative suitability for long-term use. They have associated risks as well, including cardiac conduction problems and greater potential lethality with overdose. They also have the potential to exacerbate PLMS; this fact serves to emphasize the importance of accurate initial assessment. It should be remembered that tricyclics are not hypnotics and that the mechanism underlying their beneficial use in chronic insomnia remains to be elucidated.

Patients with a primary insomnia disorder will likely require long-term treatment with sedative-hypnotic agents. Definitive data about which one is best for which patient do not yet exist. Individually demonstrated efficacy, cost, and safety are all relevant considerations. It is now clear that chronic insomnia can have serious adverse effects on performance, health, and general well-being. The prevailing attitude has been that hypnotic use should be strictly limited. However, given the advent of new compounds with demonstrated efficacy and improved safety, a relevant question is whether it is ethical to withhold such treatment.

■ REFERENCES

Adam K, Tomeny M, Oswald I: Physiological and psychological differences between good and poor sleepers. J Psychiatr Res 20:301–316, 1986

Akerstedt T: Work hours and continuous monitoring of sleepiness, in Sleep, Arousal, and Performance. Edited by Broughton RJ, Ogilvie RD. Boston, MA, Birkhäuser, 1992, pp 63–72

Allen RP, Earley CJ: Augmentation of the restless legs syndrome with carbidopa/levodopa. Sleep 19:205–213, 1996

American Academy of Sleep Medicine: The International Classification of Sleep Disorders, Revised: Diagnostic and Coding Manual. Rochester, MN, American Academy of Sleep Medicine, 2000

American Psychiatric Association: Diagnostic and Statistical Manual of Mental Disorders, 4th Edition, Text Revision. Washington, DC, American Psychiatric Association, 2000

American Sleep Disorders Association: Practice parameters for the use of polysomnography in the evaluation of insomnia. Standards of Practice Committee of the American Sleep Disorders Association. Sleep 18:55–57, 1995

Ancoli-Israel S, Kripke DF, Mason W: Sleep apnea and periodic movements in an aging sample. J Gerontol 40:419–425, 1985

Ancoli-Israel S, Seifert AR, Lemon M: Thermal biofeedback and periodic movements in sleep: patients' subjective reports and a case study. Biofeedback Self Regul 11:177–188, 1986

Ancoli-Israel S, Kripke DF, Mason W: Characteristics of obstructive and central sleep apnea in the elderly: an interim report. Biol Psychiatry 22:741–750, 1987

Biological rhythms: implications for the worker (OTA-BA-463). Washington, DC, U.S. Government Printing Office, 1991, p 18

Bonnet MH, Arand DL: 24-Hour metabolic rate in insomniacs and matched normal sleepers. Sleep 18:581–588, 1995

Broughton R, Tolentino MA, Krelina M: Excessive fragmentary myoclonus in NREM sleep: a report of 38 cases. Electroencephalogr Clin Neurophysiol 61:123–133, 1985

Carskadon MA, Vieira C, Acebo C: Association between puberty and delayed phase preference. Sleep 16:258–262, 1993

Chesson A Jr, Anderson WM, Littner M, et al: Practice parameters for the nonpharmacologic treatment of chronic insomnia. An American Academy of Sleep Medicine Report. Standards of Practice Committee of the American Academy of Sleep Medicine. Sleep 22:1128–1133, 1999a

Chesson A Jr, Wise M, Davila D, et al: Practice parameters for the treatment of restless legs syndrome and periodic limb movement disorder. An American Academy of Sleep Medicine Report. Standards of Practice Committee of the American Academy of Sleep Medicine. Sleep 22:961–968, 1999b

Coleman RM, Roffwarg HP, Kennedy SJ, et al: Sleep–wake disorders based on a polysomnographic diagnosis: a national cooperative study. JAMA 247:997–1003, 1982

Czeisler CA, Moore-Ede MC, Coleman R: Rotating shift work schedules that disrupt sleep are improved by applying circadian principles. Science 217:460–463, 1982

Czeisler CA, Allan JS, Strogatz SH, et al: Bright light resets the human circadian pacemaker independent of the timing of the sleep–wake cycle. Science 233:667–671, 1986

Czeisler CA, Dumont M, Duffy JF, et al: Association of sleep–wake habits in older people with changes in output of circadian pacemaker. Lancet 340:933–936, 1992

Davila DG, Hurt RD, Offord KP, et al: Acute effects of transdermal nicotine on sleep architecture, snoring and sleep-disordered breathing in non-smokers. Am J Respir Crit Care Med 150:469–474, 1994

Earley CJ, Hecker D, Allen RP: IV iron treatment for the restless leg syndrome (RLS) (abstract). Sleep 24(suppl):A359, 2001

Eastman CI, Stewart KT, Mahoney MP, et al: Dark goggles and bright light improve circadian rhythm adaptation to night-shift work. Sleep 17:535–543, 1994

Eastman CI, Boulos Z, Terman M, et al: Light treatment for sleep disorders: consensus report, VI: shift work. J Biol Rhythms 10:157–164, 1995

Gordon NP, Cleary PD, Parker CE, et al: The prevalence and health impact of shiftwork. Am J Public Health 76:1225–1228, 1986

Hajak G, Rodenbeck A, Staedt J, et al: Nocturnal plasma melatonin levels in patients suffering from chronic primary insomnia. J Pineal Res 19:116–122, 1995

Hauri PJ, Percy L, Hellekson C, et al: The treatment of psychophysiological insomnia with biofeedback: a replication study. Biofeedback Self Regul 7:223–235, 1983

Healey ES, Kales A, Monroe LJ, et al: Onset of insomnia: role of life-stress events. Psychosom Med 43:439–451, 1981

Hering W, Allan K, Earley C, et al: The treatment of restless legs syndrome and periodic limb movement disorder. Sleep 22:970–999, 1999

Jacobson JH, Rosenberg RS, Huttenlocher PR, et al: Familial nocturnal cramping. Sleep 9:54–60, 1986

Kayumov L, Brown G, Jindal R, et al: A randomized, double-blind, placebo-controlled crossover study of the effects of exogenous melatonin on delayed sleep phase syndrome. Psychosom Med 63:40–48, 2001

Lamarche CH, Ogilvie RD: Electrophysiological changes during the sleep onset period of psychophysiological insomniacs, psychiatric insomniacs, and normal sleepers. Sleep 20:724–733, 1997

Lugaresi E, Cirignotta F, Coccagna G, et al: Nocturnal myoclonus and restless leg syndrome, in Advances in Neurology (Series Vol 43). Edited by Fahn S. New York, Raven, 1986, pp 295–307

Mendelson WB: Insomnia and related sleep disorders. Psychiatr Clin North Am 16:841–851, 1993

Monroe LJ: Psychological and physiological differences between good and poor sleepers. J Abnorm Psychol 72:255–264, 1967

Myers BA, Klerman GL, Hartmann E: Nocturnal cataclysms with myoclonus: a new side effect of clomipramine. Am J Psychiatry 143:1490–1491, 1986

Ozaki N, Iwata T, Itoh A, et al: Body temperature monitoring in subjects with delayed sleep phase syndrome. Neuropsychobiology 20:174–177, 1988

Pasternak RE, Reynolds CR, Houck PR, et al: Sleep in bereavement-related depression during and after pharmacotherapy with nortriptyline. J Geriatr Psychiatry Neurol 7:69–73, 1994

Phillips BA, Danner FJ: Cigarette smoking and sleep disturbance. Arch Intern Med 155:734–737, 1995

Prosise GL, Bonnet MH, Berry RB, et al: Effects of abstinence from smoking on sleep and daytime sleepiness. Chest 105:1136–1141, 1994

Quinto C, Gellido C, Chokroverty S, et al: Posttraumatic delayed sleep phase syndrome. Neurology 54:250–252, 2000

Regestein Q, Monk TM: Delayed sleep phase syndrome: a review of its clinical aspects. Am J Psychiatry 152:602–608, 1995

Regestein Q, Dambrosia J, Hallett M, et al: Daytime alertness in patients with primary insomnia. Am J Psychiatry 150:1529–1534, 1993

Reynolds G, Blake DR, Pall HS, et al: Restless leg syndrome and rheumatoid arthritis. BMJ (Clinical Research Edition) 292:639–660, 1986

Sack RL, Brandes RW, Kendall AR, et al: Entrainment of free-running rhythms by melatonin in blind people. N Engl J Med 343:1070–1077, 2000

Scott AJ: Shift work and health. Prim Care 27:1057–1079, 2000

Shibui K, Uchiyama M, Okawa M: Melatonin rhythms in delayed sleep phase syndrome. J Biol Rhythms 14:72–76, 1999

Spielman AJ, Saskin P, Thorpy MJ: Treatment of chronic insomnia by restriction of time in bed. Sleep 10:45–56, 1987

Spillane JD, Nethan PW, Kelly PE, et al: Painful legs and moving toes. Brain 94:541–546, 1971

Terman M, Lewy AJ, Dijk D-J, et al: Light treatment for sleep disorders: consensus report, IV: sleep phase and duration disturbances. J Biol Rhythms 10:135–146, 1995

Ware JC: Tricyclic antidepressants in the treatment of insomnia. J Clin Psychiatry 44:25–28, 1983

Wechsler LR, Stakes JW, Shahani BT, et al: Periodic leg movements of sleep (nocturnal myoclonus): an electrophysiological study. Ann Neurol 19:168–173, 1986

Wetter DW, Fiore MC, Baker TB, et al: Tobacco withdrawal and nicotine replacement influence objective measures of sleep. J Consult Clin Psychol 63:658–667, 1995

White DP: Central sleep apnea. Med Clin North Am 9:1205–1219, 1985

EXCESSIVE SLEEPINESS DISORDERS

■ EVALUATION OF EXCESSIVE DAYTIME SLEEPINESS

Excessive daytime sleepiness (EDS) is a relatively common complaint, found in 1% of inpatients and more than 4% of industrial workers. EDS has a wide spectrum of presentation, ranging from mild sleepiness, to unrecognized episodes of "microsleeps," to uncontrollable sleep attacks. Manifestation of excessive sleepiness may vary in severity from minor decrements in performance at school or at work to catastrophic industrial or motor vehicle accidents. The Three Mile Island, Chernobyl, Bhopal, and NASA Challenger disasters all involved sleep disturbances or sleep deprivation. True EDS symptoms must be differentiated from fatigue, tiredness, and lack of motivation, which are also quite common and often associated with depression and various insomnias.

EDS is rarely found in preadolescent children, but when present it must be investigated seriously as a possible indicator of a sleep apnea disorder. Significant increases in EDS may accompany adolescence, at which point EDS may be secondary to insufficient nocturnal sleep or may herald the emergence of more serious problems such as narcolepsy, depression, or sleep apnea. College students and young adults often complain of EDS, but poor sleep habits and insufficient nocturnal sleep are often the culprits. In adults, EDS symptoms may result from a variety of causes, ranging from medical disorders to poor sleep habits. EDS symptoms must be considered serious and be evaluated both quickly and comprehensively, because they may represent potentially serious medical disorders in need of treatment and because the symptoms themselves can have serious consequences. Frequent causes of EDS are listed in Table 4–1.

TABLE 4–1. **Frequent causes of excessive daytime sleepiness**

Sleep apnea and other sleep-related breathing disorders
Narcolepsy
Primary hypersomnia (idiopathic hypersomnia)
Psychiatric disorders
Periodic limb movement disorder
Chronic use of drugs or alcohol
Other medical disorders
Periodic hypersomnias (Kleine-Levin syndrome and menstruation-associated hypersomnia)
Insufficient sleep
Sleep–wake cycle disorder
Long sleeper

The evaluation of EDS begins with a good history of daytime function. The clinician should ask the patient about alertness throughout the day, emphasizing times when sleepiness may be most likely, such as in boring, sedentary situations. The clinician should explore the use of naps (frequency, duration, and effect on alertness). He or she should ask the patient specific questions about uncontrollable sleepiness when engaging in activities such as eating, walking, talking, driving, or operating equipment. The clinician must examine subtle diminution in alertness manifested by decrements in performance at work, difficulty with memory, or confusional spells. The use of caffeine and other stimulants (including over-the-counter products) may indicate the presence of an underlying EDS disorder. All medications used should be reviewed with regard to their possible sedative or stimulant side effects. In addition, the onset, duration, and possible periodicity of daytime sleepiness are of diagnostic value. The clinician should obtain a family history with regard to symptoms of excessive somnolence and cataplexy.

Complaints of EDS may first emerge in children when they fall asleep in school or fail to pay attention in the classroom. Such children are often first thought to be lazy. Again, a complete description of the symptoms, perhaps obtained from the teacher, is important, as well as appropriate medical and family history.

The degree of daytime alertness may be subjectively quantified with rating scales such as the Stanford Sleepiness Scale (Hoddes et al. 1973) and the Epworth Sleepiness Scale (Johns 1991) or objectively quantified with the Multiple Sleep Latency Test (MSLT), as described in Chapter 1.

Figure 4–1 is a decision tree intended as a guide for the evaluation of an EDS complaint. This decision tree suggests that insufficient sleep resulting from either an insomnia disorder or poor sleep hygiene or habits should be considered first. If these causes seem unlikely, then the clinician should explore EDS secondary to a sleep-related breathing disorder, narcolepsy, or a psychiatric disorder, as well as less common causes of EDS. The evaluation process should not stop with the first evidence suggesting an etiology, because more than one cause may be operative (e.g., obstructive sleep apnea in a patient with previously undiagnosed narcolepsy). During the initial evaluation, the clinician should consider all possibilities.

In most patients with an EDS complaint, a polysomnogram and the MSLT will be required as part of the diagnostic evaluation. Exceptions would be those patients whose complaints seem clearly related to insufficient nocturnal sleep, poor sleep habits, or a psychiatric disorder that can be separately treated. In these cases, the effects of treatment of the underlying disorder on the EDS complaint should be monitored. If the EDS symptoms diminish when the underlying disorder is treated, further sleep workup may not be needed. If these symptoms do not decrease, a polysomnogram and MSLT may still be needed.

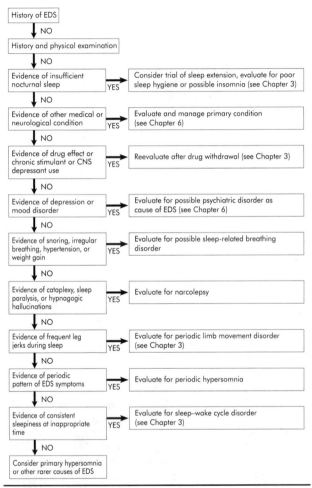

FIGURE 4–1. **Decision tree for evaluation of excessive daytime sleepiness (EDS) complaint.**

CNS=central nervous system.

■ NARCOLEPSY

Presenting Complaints

- EDS
- Episodes of irresistible sleepiness
- Paroxysmal muscle weakness, often elicited by emotion or surprise (cataplexy)
- Temporary inability to initiate motor movement before sleep or on awakening (sleep paralysis)
- Hypnagogic hallucinations
- Automatic behavior
- Disturbed nocturnal sleep

Clinical Presentation

EDS, the hallmark of narcolepsy, typically begins between ages 10 and 30 years. EDS may initially be manifested as a greater tendency to fall asleep in situations in which many people may fall asleep, such as during classes or lectures, after eating, while riding in cars, while in warm environments, or situations in which a person is excessively tired. The pathological aspect of narcolepsy may become more apparent after detection of frequent dozing off in unusual circumstances such as while standing up, walking, or doing physical exercise or painful or typically stimulating activities.

Typical warning signals of the onset of a "sleep attack" may be tiredness, heaviness of limbs, an inability to keep open or focus the eyes, loss of neck muscle tone (or "head bobbing"), and occasionally hypnagogic hallucinations. Most sleep episodes come on gradually with enough warning for the narcoleptic person to get into a safe position or pull a car to the side of the road before having an accident. Eventually, the narcoleptic patient may succumb to sleep, which often lasts 10–30 minutes and will most frequently be followed by a short period of improved alertness and a feeling of being refreshed. The most dangerous symptom of narcolepsy is the sudden onset of sleep with no warning, which can result in accidents while driving or working. It has been reported that 48% of narcoleptic individuals have fallen asleep while driving (Parkes 1983).

The frequency of daytime naps varies widely among narcoleptic patients but is generally reported to be in the range of one to eight per day. In addition to these irresistible periods of sleep, narcoleptic persons will frequently have very brief microsleeps throughout the day, as well as periods of subwakefulness or significantly impaired alertness.

Evidence indicates that some narcoleptic patients have a rhythmicity to their tendency toward sleepiness during the day that may be similar to the approximately 90-minute periodicity of rapid eye movement (REM) sleep during nocturnal sleep. For many of these individuals, it is easier to fight off early morning attacks of sleepiness; as the day proceeds, they may be less and less able to avoid napping.

The classic narcoleptic tetrad is EDS, cataplexy, sleep paralysis, and hypnagogic hallucinations. It is estimated that only 10%–15% of narcoleptic patients have the full tetrad of symptoms, and members of the same family can have different traits within the tetrad (Yoss and Daly 1957) (see Table 4–2).

TABLE 4–2.   **Frequency of symptoms in narcolepsy**

Symptom	Frequency (%)
Excessive daytime sleepiness	100
Cataplexy	70
Hypnagogic hallucinations	30
Sleep paralysis	25

Note.   *All* symptoms occur in only about 10%–15% of patients.
Source.   Sours 1963; Yoss and Daly 1957.

Cataplexy is the sudden partial or complete loss of muscle tone in response to abrupt emotional stimuli such as laughter, anger, surprise, or joy. Frequently, loss of muscle tone is confined to the face, neck, and limbs, but a generalized cataplexy with complete skeletal muscle atonia and paralysis occasionally occurs. During the episode, the person has loss of tendon reflexes, occasionally a positive Babinski sign, and loss of pupillary light reaction. Usually, these episodes last no more than a few seconds and do not result in injury to the patient or loss of consciousness. If they are prolonged (i.e., up to a minute long), full-blown REM sleep will ensue.

Cataplectic attacks can vary in frequency from once in many years to 15–20 times per day. Approximately 70% of all narcoleptic patients experience occasional cataplexy; 10%–20% of patients have improvement over time, and many can learn to diminish the frequency of episodes by avoiding sudden excitement or by tensing muscles during situations that might trigger the cataplexy (Sours 1963; Yoss and Daly 1957). Cataplexy most often appears several years after the onset of EDS, with individual case onsets reported as much as 30 years later.

Sleep paralysis occurs in about 25% of narcoleptic individuals (Sours 1963; Yoss and Daly 1957). A typical patient will complain that once or twice per week, usually at the time of sleep onset or awakening, he or she is paralyzed except for respiratory and eye musculature, but mental alertness is maintained. The paralysis seems to be terminated by noises, external stimuli, or the patient falling asleep.

Hypnagogic hallucinations are vivid auditory, somasthetic, or visual dreamlike hallucinations that usually occur at sleep onset. These episodes, which typically last only a few minutes, often accompany sleep paralysis and occur in about 30% of narcoleptic individuals (Sours 1963; Yoss and Daly 1957). Hypnagogic hallucinations and sleep paralysis are not unique to narcolepsy, however, as described in Chapter 5.

Automatic behavior is present in 20%–40% of narcoleptic individuals (Sours 1963; Yoss and Daly 1957). These episodes often consist of memory lapses, repetitive meaningless behaviors, and spoken phrases or written sentences totally out of previous context. Automatic behavior frequently occurs while driving, with long periods apparently forgotten or with travel to an unintended destination for no apparent reason. Such episodes can also contribute to illegal driving behavior, car accidents, and poor work performance.

Sleep drunkenness consists of mental clouding and confusion for the first 30–60 minutes after morning awakening. This symptom is a characteristic in approximately 10% of narcoleptic individuals.

The nocturnal sleep in most narcoleptic patients is often significantly disrupted. They are prone to frequent nocturnal spontaneous arousals as well as a greater incidence of periodic limb movement disorder (PLMD) and sleep apnea.

Although remissions have been reported, the overall course of the illness tends to show clinical stability or mild deterioration. There is no cure for narcolepsy, but in most cases the symptoms can be adequately managed.

Incidence

The prevalence of narcolepsy has been estimated to be between 0.02% and 0.07% of the population (Bixler et al. 1979). One-third of all narcoleptic individuals have positive family histories, and relatives of narcoleptic persons have a 60-fold greater chance of developing narcolepsy themselves.

Etiology and Pathophysiology

The primary daytime symptoms of narcolepsy can be thought of as both the problems of maintaining normal alertness (manifested by excessive sleepiness) and the problems with abnormal intrusion of REM sleep physiology into wakefulness (e.g., cataplexy). REM sleep physiology includes a descending inhibition of neuronal input to striated muscle. When this occurs during wakefulness, it results in the abrupt loss of muscle tone seen in cataplexy and sleep paralysis. Hypnagogic hallucinations appear related to the dreamlike mentation accompanying REM sleep occurring immediately after wakefulness.

These symptoms suggest that the processes that control sleep (perhaps both REM and non-REM) are involved in the pathophysiology of narcolepsy. Narcolepsy studies conducted in dogs have shown that the central α_1 receptor is involved in cataplexy. Administration of prazosin, a selective α_1-receptor blocker, worsens cataplexy, whereas treatment with the α_1 agonist methoxamine ameliorates it.

Nearly all narcoleptic individuals have been found to have the major histocompatibility antigen HLADQB1*0602/DQA1*0102. This has been found in studies involving Caucasian American, African American, and Japanese populations (Mignot et al. 1995). The familial incidence of narcolepsy, along with this association of narcolepsy with HLADQB1*0602/DQA1*0102, suggests that a genetic defect that manifests itself as either a neurochemical or possibly an immunological defect occurs in narcoleptic individuals.

Recent findings indicate that abnormalities of the hypocretin system in the central nervous system (CNS) occur in individuals with narcolepsy. Hypocretins, also known as orexins, are neuropeptides found in hypothalamic neurons. Hypocretin-containing neurons project widely throughout the CNS; there are axonal projections to the locus coeruleus, raphe nuclei, medullary reticular formation, and thalamus, areas known to be involved in sleep–wake regulation. Deficiency of hypocretin in cerebrospinal fluid has been demonstrated in living patients with narcolepsy. Brains of narcoleptic patients have a reduced number of hypocretin neurons at autopsy. Canine narcolepsy has been shown to be associated with a mutation of the gene coding for one hypocretin receptor. These findings suggest that abnormalities of the hypocretin system may play a central role in the pathophysiology of narcolepsy. Autoradiographic studies of narcoleptic brains have also shown increases in dopamine receptors (D_1 and D_2) and α_2 receptors in various regions (caudate nucleus and putamen) (Aldrich et al. 1993; Thannickal et al. 2000).

These findings, along with data from narcoleptic canine studies showing increased concentrations of dopamine, norepinephrine, and epinephrine, suggest that abnormalities in hypocretin, cholinergic, and monoamine systems may play an integral part in narcolepsy.

In addition to idiopathic cases of narcolepsy, events such as head trauma (Lankford et al. 1994), infections, and tumors cause some individuals to become symptomatic. It is unclear whether these events trigger narcolepsy in individuals who have a genetic predisposition or whether the events are coincidental or represent a completely different etiology.

Laboratory Findings

Narcolepsy is one of the few sleep disorders for which sleep laboratory findings are specific—both excessive sleepiness and a greater-than-normal tendency for REM sleep. The MSLT most often shows an abnormally short mean sleep latency (5 minutes or less) for five nap periods. This finding, in addition to the presence of two or more sleep-onset REM sleep periods (REM sleep within 10 minutes of sleep onset) on the MSLT, is considered diagnostic of narcolepsy. Typical MSLT findings for a group of narcoleptic patients are shown in Figure 4–2. A nocturnal polysomnogram should precede the MSLT to ensure that the previous night's sleep was not severely abnormal (e.g., severe sleep apnea). Moderate sleep disturbances are commonly found on the preceding night's polysomnogram, in the form of frequent limb movements, mild sleep apnea, and frequent awakenings. Abnormally short REM latencies will not necessarily be seen on the polysomnogram.

Differential Diagnosis

Narcolepsy is strongly suggested by the presence of the narcoleptic tetrad, especially EDS and cataplexy (Table 4–3), and further supported by a positive family history. The diagnosis can be confirmed by an MSLT with an average sleep latency of less than 5 minutes and two sleep-onset REM sleep periods and can be further supported by the presence of HLADQB1*0602/DQA1*0102 antigen. The presence of a borderline MSLT result should not eliminate the diagnosis of narcolepsy if this disorder is still strongly suspected clinically. The onset of the symptoms of narcolepsy can vary, and a distribution of sleep latencies and presence of sleep-onset REM sleep periods among narcoleptic individuals are likely. Narcoleptic patients who have negative MSLT results frequently show positive findings on subsequent studies.

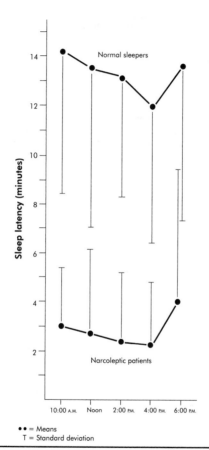

FIGURE 4–2. **Typical Multiple Sleep Latency Test (MSLT) findings for group of narcoleptic patients.**

Narcoleptic patients have shorter sleep latencies than do normal sleepers on each of the five naps constituting the MSLT.

Source. Reprinted from Hauri P: *The Sleep Disorders.* Kalamazoo, MI, Upjohn, 1982, p. 55. Used with permission of Pharmacia Corporation.

TABLE 4–3. **DSM-IV-TR diagnostic criteria for narcolepsy**

A. Irresistible attacks of refreshing sleep that occur daily over at least 3 months.

B. The presence of one or both of the following:

    (1) cataplexy (i.e., brief episodes of sudden bilateral loss of muscle tone, most often in association with intense emotion)

    (2) recurrent intrusions of elements of rapid eye movement (REM) sleep into the transition between sleep and wakefulness, as manifested by either hypnopompic or hypnagogic hallucinations or sleep paralysis at the beginning or end of sleep episodes

C. The disturbance is not due to the direct physiological effects of a substance (e.g., a drug of abuse, a medication) or another general medical condition.

The clinician must remember that it is not uncommon for individuals to feign narcolepsy to obtain stimulants. For this reason, urine drug screens in suspected individuals may be necessary to ensure that sleep latency is not shortened by the abuse of sedatives or withdrawal from stimulants. Similarly, even though the presence of cataplexy is pathognomonic for the diagnosis of narcolepsy, this symptom is self-reported. Thus, the diagnosis should be confirmed by sleep laboratory studies for protection of both patient and physician.

Severe visual imagery in some narcoleptic patients can be misinterpreted as schizophrenic hallucinatory phenomena, and misdiagnosis has been noted to occur (Reite 1998).

Other causes of EDS, listed in Table 4–1, should be excluded before a final diagnosis of narcolepsy is made. Of course, a patient may have more than one cause of EDS, and this would have treatment implications.

Treatment

Comprehensive therapy for the narcoleptic patient includes both behavioral and pharmacological components (see Table 4–4). The

---

TABLE 4–4.   **Treatment of narcolepsy**

Behavioral

Maximal sleep hygiene

Scheduled naps

Education for patient, family, teachers, employers

Pharmacological

Stimulants to control excessive daytime sleepiness

Anticataplexy medication if necessary

Treatment of associated symptoms such as disrupted nocturnal sleep or
  depression if necessary

---

clinician must keep in mind the chronicity of the disorder as well as
its pervasive effects on occupational, emotional, social, and physical functioning. Of prime importance should be helping to prevent
the patient from falling asleep while driving or working in a dangerous setting. Practice parameters for the treatment of narcolepsy
were recently updated (Littner et al. 2001a).

Behavioral Components

- *Optimize sleep hygiene to maximize the quality and quantity of
  nocturnal sleep* (see Chapter 3 for details). In narcoleptic patients, it is especially important to strive for achievement of a
  restful night's sleep by maintaining regular bedtime and awakening time; having a bedroom that is cool, comfortable, and free
  of excessive noise, light, or distraction; and taking stimulant
  doses early enough in the day to avoid interference with sleep
  onset. Alcohol should be avoided, and sedatives or tranquilizers
  should be used only as specifically warranted for treatment of
  concomitant sleep problems such as PLMD or poorly consoli-
  dated nocturnal sleep. Exercise can both increase the depth of
  nocturnal sleep and provide a temporary way to overcome
  drowsiness.
- *Instruct the patient to take brief (15–30 minutes), regularly
  scheduled daytime naps.* Naps have been shown to be an effec-

tive adjunctive treatment for sleepiness in narcoleptic patients.

- *Educate the patient and the patient's family, teachers, and employers regarding the treatment and the natural history of this illness.* A chronic illness can be very discouraging and disruptive for both patient and family. An employer or teacher especially must be aware of the nature of the illness and specifically the need to take daytime naps. The physician may need to collaborate with the employer to explain both the napping and the need for stimulant medication.

Pharmacological Components

The following pharmacological components are designed to target daytime sleepiness, cataplexy, and associated symptoms. Daytime sleepiness is generally managed with stimulant medication, either an indirect sympathomimetic or modafinil (see Table 4–5). The indirect sympathomimetics (amphetamine, methamphetamine, methylphenidate, and pemoline) appear to cause psychomotor stimulation by enhancing dopaminergic activity. Although modafinil's mechanism of action is unclear, the drug has direct α_1 noradrenergic agonist properties and appears to have fewer side effects than the indirect sympathomimetics. There also is evidence that modafinil may activate hypocretin neurons, which are now suspected of playing a role in the pathophysiology of narcolepsy. Because there is marked individual difference in tolerance and efficacy of these drugs, initiating therapy with the drugs that have the fewest side effects (modafinil or methylphenidate) is suggested. Modafinil is generally well tolerated, although headaches are reported.

Methylphenidate is commonly used in narcolepsy. Although most patients consider it to be less alerting than dextroamphetamine, it tends to be better tolerated, with less anorexia, less tachycardia, and fewer increases in blood pressure.

Dextroamphetamine and methamphetamine lead to the greatest improvement in alertness. The only study to date showing near normalization of alertness as measured by the MSLT found that

TABLE 4–5.	Pharmacological treatment of narcolepsy	
	Typical starting dosage (mg/day)	Usual dose (mg)
Stimulants		
Modafinil	100–200	400
Methylphenidate	5–20	≤100
Dextroamphetamine	5–15	≤100
Methamphetamine	5–15	≤80
Anticataplectic agents		
Protriptyline	5	≤30
Imipramine	10	≤100
Desipramine	10	≤100
Fluoxetine	20	≤60

methamphetamine, at doses of 40–60 mg, improved mean sleep latency from 4.3 minutes to 9.3 minutes on that test (Mitler et al. 1993). High doses of these agents have been associated with hallucinations and psychosis.

Pemoline is a relatively mild stimulant that has been associated with significant hepatic damage. Therefore, use of this agent is no longer recommended.

A number of other agents have been used to improve alertness (e.g., codeine, γ-hydroxybutyrate, and selegiline), but their effectiveness has not been consistently substantiated with double-blind evaluations.

Treatment of cataplexy, sleep paralysis, and hypnagogic hallucinations typically involves the use of REM-suppressing drugs. Agents that block the reuptake of norepinephrine, such as the tricyclic antidepressants protriptyline or imipramine, have been effectively used, but side effects may be limiting. Serotonin reuptake inhibitors such as fluoxetine may be helpful, but relatively high doses may be necessary. Monoamine oxidase inhibitors, clonidine, γ-hydroxybutyrate, and viloxazine have been used in difficult cases of cataplexy.

Treatment of disturbed nocturnal sleep can be problematic. If other primary sleep disorders (e.g., obstructive apnea or PLMD) are evident on the polysomnogram, specific treatment for those entities should be considered (e.g., nasal continuous positive airway pressure [CPAP] therapy or administration of a dopaminergic agent). If only fragmented nocturnal sleep is evident, γ-hydroxybutyrate or a hypnotic agent can be used. Unfortunately, improved nocturnal sleep continuity does not lead to improved daytime alertness.

A general strategy is to have the patient take stimulants in divided doses, with either the majority or half of the total dose after rising in the morning and the second dose after a brief nap around noon. Anticataplexy medication can be taken in the morning if it has stimulant properties (e.g., fluoxetine or protriptyline) or at bedtime if it has sedative properties (imipramine or desipramine) (see Table 4–5) ("Practice Parameters for the Use of Stimulants in the Treatment of Narcolepsy" 1994).

Some narcoleptic patients experience a significant degree of depression along with their illness. It is important to give the patient an opportunity to talk about the effects that the illness has on his or her life, and this may best be done by arranging for formal psychotherapy. If tricyclic antidepressants are necessary at full doses, the clinician must ensure that the sedative effects do not interfere with control of the daytime sleepiness of the narcolepsy.

■ HYPERSOMNIA DUE TO SLEEP-RELATED BREATHING DISORDERS

In this section, we consider primarily the sleep-related breathing disorders that result in symptoms of EDS (i.e., obstructive sleep apnea and related disorders). These conditions can be viewed as manifestations of ever-increasing resistance to airflow in the upper airway (see Figure 4–3). At one end of the continuum is an upper airway that is always patent in all stages of sleep. At the other end is an upper airway that frequently collapses (obstructive apnea), which causes severe decreases in oxygen saturation, hemodynamic

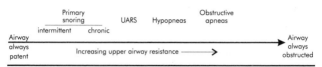

FIGURE 4–3. **Progression of findings in obstructive breathing disorders of sleep.**

UARS=upper airway resistance syndrome.

effects, and sleep fragmentation. Between these points, an individual may have primary snoring (without evidence of sleep disruption or overt airway obstruction); snoring associated with sleep fragmentation and EDS (without overt airway obstruction or oxygen desaturation), known as *upper airway resistance syndrome* (UARS); and sleep-related hypopneas associated with fragmented sleep and oxygen desaturation. Symptoms of chronic obstructive pulmonary disease (COPD) can be significantly exacerbated during sleep. Central sleep apnea, which usually presents as insomnia, is discussed in Chapter 3.

Presenting Complaints

- EDS
- Snoring, often heavy, sometimes followed by a resuscitative snort
- Restless sleep
- Morning headaches
- Depression, impaired memory and concentration, and personality change
- Impotence
- Enuresis
- Decline in school performance, in children

Clinical Presentation

Although patients with sleep apnea usually have EDS, the amount of sleepiness varies greatly among individuals and frequently is minimized. Excessive sleepiness can be totally denied or may be so severe that it impairs the patient's ability to work or drive. Persons with obstructive sleep apnea are at increased risk for motor vehicle accidents. The naps that apneic patients take generally are not very refreshing.

Persons with sleep apnea generally snore, often so loudly that it is disruptive to others sleeping in the same household. Bed partners frequently note that the patient has repetitive episodes of gradually increasing snoring, followed by a silent pause and then by a loud gasp or inspiratory snort. Violent body movements sometimes accompany this resumption of airflow. The patient with obstructive apnea usually is unaware of any difficulty breathing or of the excessive body movements. Additional complaints include morning headaches, restless sleep, and a sore throat on rising.

Psychiatric symptoms, including depression or evidence of memory impairment, may be the presenting symptoms of sleep apnea. Impotence, nocturnal seizures, and enuresis are less commonly seen. More disturbing presentations of sleep apnea syndromes include automobile or machine accidents caused by falling asleep. In children, a decline in school performance (which may be inappropriately attributed to laziness) may be a presenting symptom.

Approximately 50% of adults with obstructive sleep apnea have concurrent hypertension. Approximately 70% of patients with sleep apnea are at least 20% overweight (Guilleminault 1987; Guilleminault et al. 1993). In addition, a neck circumference greater than 16.75 inches (measured at the cricothyroid membrane) is predictive of obstructive sleep apnea.

Individuals with alveolar hypoventilation, in whom a history of heavy snoring and restless sleep may be absent, may also complain of EDS. Other medical conditions that may impair ventilation, such as poliomyelitis, myotonic dystrophy, obesity, and thoracic wall abnormalities, may be present in such patients.

Patients with primary pulmonary diseases such as COPD or cystic fibrosis can have episodes of hypoxemia and/or obstructive apnea when sleeping. Patients with reactive airway disease often complain of increased wheezing, coughing, or shortness of breath during the night. They may have disrupted sleep with frequent prolonged arousals and also may complain of daytime fatigue and sleepiness.

Incidence

Sleep apnea has been estimated to occur in 2%–4% of the general population (Young et al. 1993). In addition, it is estimated that 19% of women and 30% of men are chronic heavy snorers. Sleep apnea can occur in all age groups and both sexes but is most common in middle-aged men.

Etiology and Pathophysiology

Apnea

The process of ventilation is based on air flowing down a gradient of pressure. During inspiration, the diaphragm and chest wall muscles generate a large negative intrapleural pressure. This negative pressure causes expansion of the lung parenchyma and is transmitted to the different-sized airways. The patency of the oropharyngeal airway depends on pharyngeal dilators to counteract the large negative pressure generated during inspiration. A complex neuromuscular mechanism involving the soft palate, the pharyngeal walls, and the tongue is activated in a phasic fashion to maintain airway patency. Processes that decrease this neuromuscular activity, such as the muscular hypotonia characteristic of sleep, can cause oropharyngeal airway collapse. The fact that not everyone who sleeps, and thus develops oropharyngeal hypotonia, has upper airway collapse suggests that coexisting conditions must be present. Current evidence suggests that most patients with sleep apnea have a congenitally small oropharyngeal airway. Other more obvious causes of airway obstruction (e.g., micrognathia, retrognathia, adenotonsillar hypertrophy, nasal obstruction, a large uvula, macroglossia, or malignancy) can also contribute to obstructive apnea. It appears that in many patients, muscle hypotonia in conjunction with a narrowed airway permits the obstruction to occur.

In children, obstructive apnea is most often secondary to enlargement of tonsils, adenoids, or other lymphoid tissue in the oropharynx. However, craniofacial abnormalities such as mandibular hypoplasia can result in obstructive apnea.

The consequences of repetitive episodes of apnea fall into two general categories: medical effects and the effects on sleep itself. Cessation of airflow can lead to oxygen desaturation. The degree of the desaturation depends on the duration of the respiratory event, the oxygen saturation at the beginning of the event, and the lung volume at the time of the event. Oxygen desaturation is most severe when the apneic event is very long, when the baseline oxygen saturation is already low (i.e., on the steep portion of the oxyhemoglobin dissociation curve), and when the patient has a low lung volume.

Systemic and pulmonary artery pressures increase during apneic events, and repetitive apneic events can cause a stepwise increase in both of these pressures. Once airflow is resumed, these pressures usually return to normal. Obstructive sleep apnea in an individual with normal waking pO_2 measurements is not generally believed to be a cause of significant, persistent pulmonary artery hypertension (Chaouat et al. 1996). Some data indicate that patients with essential hypertension and no specific sleep complaints may have a high incidence (about 30%) of unsuspected sleep apnea (Williams et al. 1985). This finding suggests that sleep apnea may be a contributory factor in chronic systemic hypertension. The repetitive apneic episodes may induce diurnal hypertension via an increase in sympathetic tone. Cardiac dysrhythmias have been noted to occur with respiratory events. The most common finding is sinus variability with repetitive episodes of relative bradycardia (during the obstruction), followed by an increase in heart rate (during the resumption of airflow)—the so-called bradytachycardia. Other, less common, dysrhythmias include sinus arrest, atrioventricular blocks, ventricular ectopy, and ventricular tachycardia. The frequency of dysrhythmias decreases with adequate treatment of the apnea.

Sleep apnea can also have severely disruptive effects on sleep itself. The termination of a respiratory event often requires a partial arousal from sleep. As a result, sleep for an apneic patient may be quite fragmented, consisting of short periods of light sleep interrupted by frequent arousals. These cortical arousals are often accompanied by increased sympathetic nervous system activity and an increase in skeletal muscle activity manifested by muscle jerks and more complete body movements, described as "restless" sleep. This sleep fragmentation is likely a major contributor to the development of daytime sleepiness.

Primary Pulmonary Disorders

Patients with primary pulmonary disorders such as COPD or cystic fibrosis, especially those with CO_2 retention (i.e., the "blue bloater"), often have transient episodes of severe nocturnal hypoxemia. Such patients depend more than healthy individuals on the accessory muscles of respiration for their ventilation. During REM sleep, the hypotonia of the intercostal and accessory muscles may lead to smaller tidal volumes and decreased minute ventilation. Functional residual capacity is also reduced during REM sleep. Ventilation-perfusion mismatching during REM sleep also has been hypothesized to contribute to oxygen desaturation. Cardiac arrhythmias and increased pulmonary artery pressure have been observed during these episodes of hypoxemia. A subgroup of patients with chronic pulmonary disease also have coexistent sleep apnea. The combination of these two conditions can lead to profound oxygen desaturation, especially during REM sleep. Patients with asthma may have an exaggerated nocturnal bronchoconstriction that can lead to increasing symptomatology during the night.

Laboratory Findings

An apnea is defined as the cessation of airflow for at least 10 seconds. Three types of apnea have been described: central, obstructive, and mixed. A central apnea (Figure 4–4) occurs when there is a lack of respiratory effort by the diaphragm and, hence, no airflow. An obstructive apnea (Figure 4–5) is present when respiratory effort occurs but no airflow results. A mixed apnea (Figure 4–6) is a combination of central and obstructive components, consisting of

128

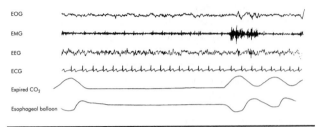

FIGURE 4–4. **Central apnea.**

Polysomnographic characteristics include absence of both airflow (indicated by no change in expired air CO_2) and respiratory effort (indicated by no change in esophageal balloon pressure).

ECG = electrocardiogram; EEG = electroencephalogram; EMG = electromyogram; EOG = electro-oculogram.

Source. Reprinted from Hauri P: *The Sleep Disorders.* Kalamazoo, MI, Upjohn, 1982, p. 56. Used with permission of Pharmacia Corporation.

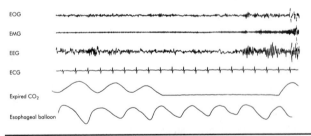

FIGURE 4–5. **Obstructive apnea.**

Polysomnographic characteristics include absence of airflow (indicated by no change in expired air CO_2) in the presence of continued respiratory effort.

ECG = electrocardiogram; EEG = electroencephalogram; EMG = electromyogram; EOG = electro-oculogram.

Source. Reprinted from Hauri P: *The Sleep Disorders.* Kalamazoo, MI, Upjohn, 1982, p. 56. Used with permission of Pharmacia Corporation.

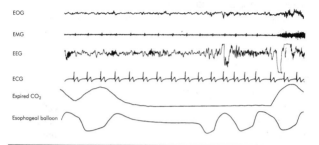

FIGURE 4–6. **Mixed apnea.**

Polysomnographic characteristics include initial absence of both airflow and effort, followed by resumption of effort but, initially, not airflow.

ECG = electrocardiogram; EEG = electroencephalogram; EMG = electromyogram; EOG = electro-oculogram.

Source. Reprinted from Hauri P: *The Sleep Disorders.* Kalamazoo, MI, Upjohn, 1982, p. 56. Used with permission of Pharmacia Corporation.

an initial central event with cessation of respiratory effort, followed by an interval of effort without airflow because the airway closed during the central event. In some patients with obstructive apnea, a "paradoxical" motion of the chest wall is seen. In these patients, the large negative intrapleural pressure created by the diaphragm causes the chest wall to retract during times of airway obstruction. The polysomnographic tracing shows a "phase reverse" of the thoracic motion in relation to abdominal motion at these times.

An apnea index (the number of apneas per 60 minutes of sleep time) of 5–8 is probably the upper limit of normal in young adults. Some studies have suggested that older patients may have as many as 17 respiratory events per hour, with only minimal decrements in daytime alertness as measured by the MSLT. Whether sleep apnea of this degree is associated with other physiological consequences is not yet known.

A decrease, but not total cessation, of airflow that lasts at least 10 seconds is termed a *hypopnea.* Both apneas and hypopneas can lead to the same end results: oxygen desaturation and arousals.

Because of these common effects, both apneas and hypopneas may be collectively described as either the respiratory disturbance index or the apnea-hypopnea index, which is equal to the sum of the apneas and hypopneas per total number of hours of sleep.

Evidence indicates that some individuals have an increase in upper airway airflow resistance *without* obvious apneas or hypopneas. These individuals exhibit increasing respiratory effort (as measured by esophageal balloon monitoring), often associated with frequent arousals (and sometimes snoring), but maintain constant airflow. Therefore, they can be viewed as "working harder" to maintain constant airflow. When this condition is associated with frequent arousals and daytime sleepiness, it is considered to be UARS (Guilleminault et al. 1993).

Sleep architecture is often abnormal in patients with obstructive sleep apnea or UARS. Typically, a polysomnogram shows fragmented sleep (composed mostly of Stage I and Stage II sleep) with frequent arousals and awakenings. The amount of Stage III, Stage IV, and REM sleep recorded is decreased. In addition, cardiac dysrhythmias, leg jerks, and body movements are noted. An MSLT done the day after a polysomnogram can help quantify the severity of EDS in patients with obstructive sleep apnea.

Patients with sleep-related hypoxemia due to nonapneic causes (e.g., COPD) have prolonged episodes of hypoxemia, especially in REM sleep. The pattern of desaturation recorded by the oximeter shows a persistently low oxygen saturation rather than a consistently changing saturation typical of repetitive apneic events.

In patients with nocturnal asthma, flow rates (measured as forced expiratory volume over a 1-second interval [i.e., peak flow rate]) that are measured throughout the night can show a decrement. These patients often complain of nocturnal wheezing and restless sleep. Their sleep is inefficient, with frequent and prolonged awakenings.

Differential Diagnosis

Nocturnal polysomnography is required for proper assessment of sleep-related breathing disorders (see Table 3–5 for DSM-IV-TR diagnostic criteria for breathing-related sleep disorders). Studies of breathing during short daytime naps are not adequate for proper diagnosis because all sleep stages may not occur. Breathing disorders are not uniformly present during sleep; they tend to wax and wane and frequently become more severe during early morning hours. Polysomnographic recording should be sufficient to assess sleep stage, respiratory effort and airflow, tibialis anterior electromyogram, oximetry, and snoring sounds. It is important to observe whether apneas are related to sleep position (e.g., supine vs. on the side). If UARS is a consideration, careful attention must be paid to evidence of episodes of increasing respiratory effort followed by cortical arousals and perhaps snoring.

EDS due to sleep apnea usually can be differentiated from EDS due to narcolepsy on clinical grounds by the age at onset (sleep apnea typically becomes symptomatic in middle age, and narcolepsy often arises during the teens or early 20s) and the lack of cataplexy, hypnagogic hallucinations, and sleep paralysis, as well as the presence of snoring, morning headaches, and naps that are not refreshing. The presence of hypertension or polycythemia also raises suspicion of a sleep-related breathing disorder.

Mood disorders (major depression and atypical depression) can present with EDS, and the sleepiness should improve with effective therapy. Because depression can also be a *symptom* of sleep apnea, careful evaluation for both problems should be considered.

Differentiating sleep apnea from other chronic causes of excessive somnolence (e.g., idiopathic hypersomnolence, chronic drug dependence, nocturnal myoclonus) often requires a nocturnal polysomnogram and other laboratory tests (e.g., thyroid function test, drug screen) and clinical evaluations (e.g., psychiatric interviews). Definitive diagnosis of nocturnal hypoxemia due to nonapneic causes begins by ruling out apnea with a polysomnogram and may then require other pulmonary function tests (e.g., basic spirometry, tests of ventilatory drive and bronchial reactivity).

Treatment

Treatments for obstructive sleep apnea are directed at improving breathing and oxygen saturation during sleep as well as reducing sleep fragmentation, with the ultimate goal of normalizing daytime alertness. Reduction of the level of snoring is frequently desired. The types of treatment available fall into three general classes: behavioral, medical, and surgical. The treatment plan for any given patient should be individualized according to the severity of the disorder and the patient's tolerance of the treatment (see Table 4–6).

If the patient has a combination of obstructive and central apneas, the obstructive events should be vigorously treated, and the central events will then often improve. Pure central apnea is rare and typically presents as insomnia rather than EDS. Treatment of central apnea insomnia is discussed further in Chapter 3.

Regardless of which treatment the clinician selects, he or she should verify its effectiveness with a repeat polysomnogram, because patients tend to overestimate their improvement.

Behavioral Techniques

Behavioral techniques include avoiding sleep deprivation, losing weight if appropriate, and using positional techniques (e.g., avoiding the supine position). If the diagnostic study finds that apneas occur only in the supine position, the patient can try to sleep on his or her side. This can be facilitated by the patient's wearing a nightshirt with back pockets containing tennis balls or other uncomfortable objects. Respiratory depressants such as alcohol and sedatives should be avoided. Smoking should be discontinued, because its irritating effect on the upper airway mucosa can lead to a worsening of sleep-related obstruction. The clinician should also counsel the patient to avoid operating motor vehicles or dangerous machinery until daytime alertness improves.

Medical Techniques

CPAP therapy is currently the most reliable form of medical treatment for obstructive sleep apnea. Air pressure is generated via a small blower unit that runs on household current and sits at the patient's bedside. The air pressure is delivered to the patient's airway via a connecting tube and mask (either a nasal mask or a full face

TABLE 4–6. Assessment and treatment plan for hypersomnia due to sleep-related breathing disorder

	Apnea-hypopnea index (respiratory events/hour)	Lowest oxygen saturation	Respiratory event-related arousal (arousals/hour)	Cardiac effects	Daytime alertness	Treatment options[a]
Snoring without apnea	<10	>90%	<5	None±hypertension	Normal	B—also earplugs for bedmate; M—oral appliance; S—palatal surgery
Upper airway resistance syndrome	<10	>90%	Often>15; may be associated with snoring	Sinus rate variability with arousals Hypertension	Impaired (mild to severe)	B—also earplugs for bedmate; M—CPAP, oral appliance; S
Obstructive apnea-hypopnea syndrome, mild	10–15	High 80% range	5–10	None or bradytachycardia with respiratory events Hypertension	Normal to impaired (mild) (MSL>9 min)	B; M—CPAP, oral appliance; S

TABLE 4-6. Assessment and treatment plan for hypersomnia due to sleep-related breathing disorder *(continued)*

	Apnea-hypopnea index (respiratory events/hour)	Lowest oxygen saturation	Respiratory event-related arousal (arousals/hour)	Cardiac effects	Daytime alertness	Treatment options[a]
Obstructive apnea-hypopnea syndrome, moderate	15–30	~80%	10–20	None or bradytachycardia with respiratory events+PVC Hypertension	Impaired (moderate) (MSL 5–9 min)	M—CPAP, oral appliance; S
Obstructive apnea-hypopnea syndrome, severe	>30	<80%	>20	None or bradytachycardia with respiratory events+PVC, AV block Hypertension	Impaired (severe) (MSL <5 min)	M—CPAP, oral appliance; S

Note. AV=atrioventricular; B=behavioral (e.g., positional changes, weight loss, avoiding alcohol); CPAP=continuous positive airway pressure; M=medical (i.e., CPAP or oral appliance); MSL=mean sleep latency on Mean Sleep Latency Test; PVC=premature ventricular contraction; S=surgical (type of surgery required is dependent on site of obstruction).
[a]A follow-up polysomnogram is suggested after treatment, to verify its effectiveness.

mask) and creates a "pneumatic splint" that holds the airway open during sleep. The air pressure necessary to maintain airway patency varies from person to person. Currently, most patients undergo a "CPAP titration" study in a sleep laboratory to determine the effective pressure, but self-titrating CPAP devices are available. Nasal CPAP therapy can lead to marked improvement in breathing, oxygen saturation, cardiac rhythm, sleep quality, and daytime alertness. However, many patients have difficulty tolerating CPAP treatment, and published compliance rates are approximately 50%–80% (Anstead et al. 1998). A similar device allows different pressures for inspiration and expiration (bilevel positive airway pressure therapy) to be selected. This device may be more comfortable for patients, but it has not been shown to improve compliance rates. Adding heated humidification to the CPAP device does improve patient compliance.

Oral appliances such as the mandibular repositioning device or tongue retaining device have been used increasingly in patients with obstructive sleep apnea and/or snoring. These appliances are fairly well tolerated but have unpredictable response rates. Therefore, a follow-up evaluation while these devices are being used is recommended (Ayas and Epstein 1998).

Supplemental oxygen may help to lessen the severity of the decreases in oxygen saturation that occur with apneas or hypopneas. Although this treatment may not improve sleep continuity, clinicians might consider it for patients who cannot tolerate other therapies. In addition, some patients who have hypoventilation in addition to obstructive apnea need to have oxygen added to the CPAP treatment.

Medications have not proved to be very useful in treating obstructive sleep apnea, although protriptyline and fluoxetine have had mild effects in some patients. Modafinil has been described as being helpful in treating residual sleepiness in patients receiving CPAP therapy (Kingshott et al. 2001).

Surgical Techniques

Various surgical treatments have been attempted for obstructive sleep apnea and snoring. Tracheostomy is the most reliable surgical approach because it bypasses the upper airway obstruction. It offers rapid improvement and typically is used in patients with severe life-threatening apnea who do not tolerate or respond to CPAP therapy. Uvulopalatopharyngoplasty has had unpredictable results, with studies suggesting success rates of approximately 50%. Practice parameters for use of laser-assisted uvulopalatoplasty have been published (Littner et al. 2001b). More extensive procedures such as maxillomandibular advancement may have more predictably successful results (Sher et al. 1996). Other surgical procedures, such as tonsillectomy, may be appropriate in certain cases, such as in children with obstructive sleep apnea who clearly have excessive lymphoid tissue and compromised airways. Practice parameters for surgical treatment of obstructive sleep apnea in adults have also been published ("Practice Parameters for the Treatment of Obstructive Sleep Apnea in Adults" 1996). Radiofrequency submucosal tissue volume reduction is a new technique that is used to try to increase upper airway size. Although it seems to be well tolerated, it has not been extensively evaluated.

Treatment of Primary Snoring

The treatment of primary snoring includes various simple behavioral measures, such as use of earplugs by the bed partner and avoidance of alcohol or the supine position. Oral appliance therapy and palatal surgery have appeared helpful to patients in studies with subjective end points. Recently, laser surgery of the soft palate (an outpatient procedure) has been used, and it can be repeated if necessary. Nasal CPAP therapy is effective in reducing snoring, but, in general, patients who have primary snoring alone do not want to use it (Hoffstein 1996).

■ NOCTURNAL HYPOXEMIA

In patients with nocturnal hypoxemia from nonapneic causes (e.g., COPD or cystic fibrosis), supplemental oxygen often improves the condition. The correct oxygen flow rate should be determined with a supervised overnight study, to avoid exacerbating hypoventilation in those patients who are oxygen sensitive. Patients who tend to hypoventilate during the day often benefit from medroxyprogesterone (20 mg three times a day) as a respiratory stimulant. Routine follow-up polysomnograms do not appear to contribute significantly to the management of COPD.

■ BRONCHOSPASM

Nocturnal symptoms in patients with bronchospasm may relate to circadian rhythm– and sleep-related changes in airway caliber as well as to environmental triggers or to the medication schedule. Bedroom exposure to allergens can heighten bronchoreactivity in some patients. Other patients who are exposed to allergens in the evening may show a delayed response 6–8 hours later, leading to bronchoconstriction during sleep. Identification and avoidance of the allergen trigger reduce symptoms. Long-acting β-agonists and sustained-release theophylline preparations can be given to achieve therapeutic medication levels throughout the night. In individuals with both obstructive sleep apnea and asthma, treatment with CPAP may lead to improvement of bronchospasm as well as elimination of obstructive respiratory events.

■ OTHER CAUSES OF EXCESSIVE DAYTIME SLEEPINESS

Sleep apnea and narcolepsy are the two leading causes of hypersomnia. Several less common causes of EDS are outlined here. (For discussion of hypersomnolence associated with psychiatric disorders, see Chapter 6.)

Somnolence Associated With Insufficient Sleep

Individuals who chronically obtain insufficient sleep as a result of occupational, educational, social, or familial demands frequently can become pathologically sleepy. These patients are often unaware that they are voluntarily depriving themselves of sleep, or they deny that this is happening.

The diagnosis of insufficient sleep is suggested when the patient's history and sleep log document chronically short sleep times. Often, marked variations occur in sleep time between weekday and weekend nights. A therapeutic trial of extending sleep time can confirm this diagnosis. Polysomnographic examinations in these patients show increased sleep efficiency and increased Stage III, Stage IV, and REM sleep when patients are permitted to sleep as long as possible. Treatment includes educating patients about their own sleep needs and encouraging consistent extension of their sleep time.

A typical long sleeper may need 9–11 hours of sleep per night. Sleep deprivation below this amount may lead to EDS. If these individuals are allowed to obtain the full amount of sleep, they should have no tendency toward EDS.

Primary Hypersomnia

Primary hypersomnia (idiopathic hypersomnia in *The International Classification of Sleep Disorders,* Revised [American Academy of Sleep Medicine 2000]) is a syndrome of persistent daytime somnolence. Patients with this disorder note an increasingly irresistible need to sleep during the day, which leads to prolonged naps. These naps are lengthy—often 60 minutes or longer—and not very refreshing. When these patients are not sleeping, they are drowsy and have difficulty concentrating. This excessive sleepiness occurs after sufficient or even increased amounts of nocturnal sleep. These patients frequently have complaints of sleep drunkenness on awakening. Diagnostic criteria are listed in Table 4–7.

In diagnosing primary hypersomnia, the clinician should identify and exclude those patients with histories of viral infections, including mononucleosis, viral pneumonia, Guillain-Barré syndrome, and encephalitis, that correspond to hypersomnia due to a medical condition. Such exclusions leave those patients with family

---

TABLE 4–7. **DSM-IV-TR diagnostic criteria for primary hypersomnia**

A. The predominant complaint is excessive sleepiness for at least 1 month (or less if recurrent) as evidenced by either prolonged sleep episodes or daytime sleep episodes that occur almost daily.

B. The excessive sleepiness causes clinically significant distress or impairment in social, occupational, or other important areas of functioning.

C. The excessive sleepiness is not better accounted for by insomnia and does not occur exclusively during the course of another Sleep Disorder (e.g., Narcolepsy, Breathing-Related Sleep Disorder, Circadian Rhythm Sleep Disorder, or a Parasomnia) and cannot be accounted for by an inadequate amount of sleep.

D. The disturbance does not occur exclusively during the course of another mental disorder.

E. The disturbance is not due to the direct physiological effects of a substance (e.g., a drug of abuse, a medication) or a general medical condition.

Specify if:

Recurrent: if there are periods of excessive sleepiness that last at least 3 days occurring several times a year for at least 2 years

---

histories of daytime somnolence (these patients may also have symptoms related to abnormal autonomic function, such as Raynaud's phenomenon, orthostatic hypotension, or syncope) and those without family histories of EDS or previous significant viral illness (i.e., an idiopathic group).

Laboratory Findings

Laboratory findings for primary hypersomnia include polysomnographic evidence of normal nocturnal sleep without evidence of breathing disorders, leg jerks, or sleep fragmentation. The MSLT usually demonstrates shortened mean sleep latency of about 5–6 minutes. If the polysomnogram indicates frequent sleep fragmentation caused by spontaneous arousals as the *only* abnormality in a patient with suspected primary hypersomnia, further monitoring with an esophageal balloon may be warranted to evaluate for possible UARS.

Differential Diagnosis

Primary hypersomnia usually can be differentiated from narcolepsy by the absence of cataplexy, hypnagogic hallucinations, and sleep paralysis. Sleep apnea is suggested by a history of snoring. A polysomnogram and the MSLT are necessary to differentiate primary hypersomnia from the other causes of EDS. Patients with primary hypersomnia do not demonstrate sleep-onset REM sleep periods on the MSLT, as is commonly seen in narcolepsy.

Treatment

Treatment of primary hypersomnia has been difficult. Typically, stimulant medication is useful, but most patients still complain of daytime sleepiness and take daily naps. Recently, modafinil has been used successfully in such patients.

Hypersomnia Associated With Drug and Alcohol Use

Patients who have hypersomnia associated with drug and alcohol use are somnolent either as a result of the direct sedating effect of a drug or as a result of drug withdrawal. These conditions are discussed in Chapter 3.

Periodic Hypersomnias

Kleine-Levin Syndrome

Kleine-Levin syndrome is an uncommon periodic hypersomnia disorder that is most common in males, often beginning in the teen years. Typically, the patient has one or more episodes yearly that are characterized by periods of excessive sleepiness that often last for weeks. During these hypersomnolent times, the patient can be aroused, but when awake, he or she is confused and agitated and has a loss of sexual inhibitions. While in this somnolent state, patients can have insatiable appetites, especially when presented with food. The patient has minimal recollection of the hypersomnolent period after the episode clears. He or she appears normal between attacks. Usually, this disorder spontaneously remits by age 40. The etiology of Kleine-Levin syndrome is unknown, but disorders of several brain regions, including the thalamus, brain stem, frontal lobes, and hypothalamus, have been suggested.

Laboratory findings.   Electroencephalographic evaluations done during the wakeful portions of a hypersomnolent episode have shown mild intermittent slowing. Nocturnal sleep has been reported to lack Stage III and Stage IV sleep. Also, shortened REM sleep latency has been reported, and even an occasional sleep-onset REM sleep period has been recorded. Although cerebrospinal fluid is usually normal in these patients, a few studies have found levels of 5-hydroxyindoleacetic acid to be increased.

Differential diagnosis.   The periodic nature of the somnolence, along with the abnormal behavior, confusion, and compulsive eating, differentiates Kleine-Levin syndrome from other common causes of excessive somnolence. The clinician should consider other psychiatric disorders (especially bipolar disorder and schizophrenia), drug-induced states, and metabolic and inflammatory disorders in the differential diagnosis.

Treatment.   Because Kleine-Levin syndrome is self-limited, many patients are not treated. Stimulant medication has been useful in treating the somnolence, but it can worsen the behavioral problems. Lithium has had some success in prophylaxis of the hypersomnolent episodes.

Menstruation-Associated Hypersomnia

Some females become periodically hypersomnolent around the time of their menses. They often act uncharacteristically (e.g., withdraw or exhibit apathy or irritability) during these somnolent times and may awaken only for bathroom visits. After menstruation, these patients resume their regular behavior and daytime alertness. The etiology is not known, but hypothalamic dysfunction is hypothesized.

Laboratory findings.   Decreased amounts of Stage III and Stage IV sleep have been noted in the few cases of this uncommon disorder that were polysomnographically evaluated.

Differential diagnosis.   The characteristic relation of the hypersomnia to the menstrual cycle differentiates this disorder from most other causes of EDS. To exclude medication-induced somnolence, the clinician must obtain a careful history regarding medications used for menstrual symptoms.

Treatment.   There have been reports of total cessation of the hypersomnia when ovulation was blocked by oral contraceptive agents.

Excessive Daytime Sleepiness Associated with Periodic Limb Movements Disorder

Patients with PLMD usually complain of insomnia but can have EDS as a symptom as well. Investigators believe that sleep fragmentation due to repetitive arousals associated with leg jerks is the mechanism producing daytime sleepiness. The patient often does not suspect PLMD, and a polysomnographic evaluation is required for diagnosis. PLMD can coexist with either narcolepsy or sleep apnea. (The diagnosis and treatment of PLMD are described in Chapter 3.)

■ REFERENCES

Aldrich MS, Hollingsworth Z, Penney JB: Autoradiographic studies of postmortem human narcoleptic brain. Neurophysiol Clin 23:35–45, 1993

American Academy of Sleep Medicine: The International Classification of Sleep Disorders, Revised: Diagnostic and Coding Manual. Rochester, MN, American Academy of Sleep Medicine, 2000

Anstead M, Phillips B, Buch K: Tolerance and intolerance to continuous positive airway pressure. Curr Opin Pulm Med 4:351–354, 1998

Ayas NT, Epstein LJ: Oral appliances in the treatment of obstructive sleep apnea and snoring. Curr Opin Pulm Med 4:355–360, 1998

Bixler E, Kales A, Soldatos C, et al: Prevalence of sleep disorders: a survey of the Los Angeles metropolitan area. Am J Psychiatry 136:1257–1262, 1979

Chaouat A, Weitzenblum E, Krieger J, et al: Pulmonary hemodynamics in the obstructive sleep apnea syndrome. Results in 220 consecutive patients. Chest 109:380–386, 1996

Guilleminault C: Obstructive sleep apnea syndrome: a review. Psychiatr Clin North Am 10:607–621, 1987

Guilleminault C, Shoohs R, Clerk A, et al: A cause of excessive daytime sleepiness: the upper airway resistance syndrome. Chest 104:781–787, 1993

Hoddes E, Zarcone V, Smythe H, et al: Quantification of sleepiness: a new approach. Psychophysiology 10:431–436, 1973

Hoffstein V: Snoring. Chest 109:201–222, 1996

Johns MW: A new method for measuring daytime sleepiness: the Epworth Sleepiness Scale. Sleep 14:540–545, 1991

Kingshott RN, Venelle M, Coleman EL, et al: Randomized, double-blind, placebo-controlled crossover trial of modafinil in the treatment of residual excessive daytime sleepiness in the sleep apnea/hypopnea syndrome. Am J Respir Crit Care Med 163:918–923, 2001

Lankford D, Wellman J, O'Hara C: Posttraumatic narcolepsy in mild to moderate closed head injury. Sleep 17:525–558, 1994

Littner M, Johnson SF, McCall WW, et al: Practice parameters for the treatment of narcolepsy: an update for 2000. Sleep 24:451–456, 2001a

Littner M, Kushida CA, Hartse K, et al: Practice parameters for the use of laser-assisted uvulopalatoplasty: an update for 2000. Sleep 24:603–619, 2001b

Mignot E, Tafti M, Dement WC, et al: Narcolepsy and immunity. Adv Immunol 5:23–37, 1995

Mitler MM, Hajdukovic R, Erman MK: Treatment of narcolepsy with methamphetamine. Sleep 16:306–317, 1993

Parkes JD: The sleepy driver, in Driving and Epilepsy and Other Causes of Impaired Consciousness. Edited by Godwin-Austen RB, Espir MLE. London, England, Royal Society of Medicine, 1983, pp 23–27

Practice parameters for the treatment of obstructive sleep apnea in adults: the efficacy of surgical modifications of the upper airway. Report of the American Sleep Disorders Association. Sleep 19:152–155, 1996

Practice parameters for the use of stimulants in the treatment of narcolepsy. Standards of Practice Committee of the American Sleep Disorders Association. Sleep 17:348–351, 1994

Reite M: Sleep disorders presenting as psychiatric disorders. Psychiatr Clin North Am 21:591–607, 1998

Sher A, Schechtman K, Piccirillo J: The efficacy of surgical modification of the upper airway in adults with obstructive sleep apnea. Sleep 19:156–177, 1996

Sours JA: Narcolepsy and other disturbances in sleep wake rhythm: a study of 115 cases with review. J Nerv Ment Dis 137:525–542, 1963

Thannickal TC, Moore RY, Nienhuis R, et al: Reduced number of hypocretin neurons in human narcolepsy. Neuron 27:469–474, 2000

Williams AJ, Houston D, Finberg S, et al: Sleep apnea syndrome and essential hypertension. Am J Cardiol 55:1019–1022, 1985

Yoss RE, Daly DD: Criteria for the diagnosis of the narcoleptic syndrome. Proceedings of the Staff Meetings of the Mayo Clinic 32:320–328,1957

Young T, Palta M, Dempsey J, et al: The occurrence of sleep disordered breathing among middle aged adults. N Engl J Med 328:1230–1235, 1993

5

PARASOMNIAS

The four general categories of parasomnias discussed in this chapter (see Table 5–1) are 1) parasomnias usually associated with rapid eye movement (REM) sleep (e.g., nightmares and REM sleep behavior disorders), 2) arousal disorders (e.g., sleepwalking and night terrors), 3) sleep–wake transition disorders, and 4) miscellaneous parasomnias unrelated to sleep stage or secondary to other organ system abnormalities that arise during sleep.

■ PARASOMNIAS ASSOCIATED WITH REM SLEEP

Nightmares

Nightmares are frightening dreams that usually occur during a long and often convoluted dream sequence that provokes intense fear or anxiety. The context of the dream often includes fear of physical danger to the dreamer but may also contain themes of personal humiliation or repetition of past trauma. A nightmare generally ends when the dreamer is fully alert, but he or she continues to have a feeling of fear or anxiety. The individual can usually recount the dream in great detail. Nightmares can occur at any time during the night, but because they usually occur in REM sleep, they are more frequent toward morning, when REM sleep periods are longer. Because of the brain's inhibition of muscle activity during REM sleep, no motor activity occurs during nightmares, except in some severe cases of posttraumatic stress disorder (PTSD). That disorder also has the ability to trigger nightmare activity in non-REM sleep (Ross et al. 1994).

TABLE 5–1. Parasomnias

Associated with REM sleep	Arousal disorders	Sleep–wake transition disorders	Secondary to specific organ system abnormalities	Miscellaneous
Nightmares	Sleepwalking	Sleep starts	**CNS parasomnias**	Nocturnal sleep–related eating disorder
Sleep paralysis	Sleep terrors	Hypnic jerks	Nocturnal seizures	Sleep bruxism
Hypnagogic hallucinations	Confusional arousal	Sensory starts	Vascular headaches	Sleep-related tonic spasms
Hypnopompic hallucinations		Sleeptalking	Exploding head syndrome	Primary snoring
REM sleep behavior disorder			Hypnic headache syndrome	Sleep drunkenness
Sleep-related impaired penile erections			Nocturnal paroxysmal dystonia	Benign neonatal sleep myoclonus
Sleep-related painful penile erections			Tinnitus	
REM sleep–related sinus arrest			**Cardiopulmonary parasomnias**	
			Cardiac arrhythmias	
			Nocturnal angina pectoris	
			Nocturnal asthma	
			Respiratory dyskinesias	
			Sleep hiccup	
			Sudden unexplained nocturnal death syndrome	

TABLE 5–1. Parasomnias *(continued)*

Associated with REM sleep	Arousal disorders	Sleep–wake transition disorders	Secondary to specific organ system abnormalities	Miscellaneous
			Gastrointestinal parasomnias Gastroesophageal reflux Sleep-related abnormal swallowing syndrome Diffuse esophageal spasm	

Note. CNS=central nervous system; REM=rapid eye movement.

Nightmares occur in all age groups but are most frequent in early childhood. Their peak incidence is at ages 3–5 years; frequency diminishes with age. Among adults, nightmares are more common in women. The small percentage who have nightmare disorder as adults tend to complain of sleep loss, daytime sleepiness, fear of falling or returning to sleep, and increases in anxiety and mood disturbances. The DSM-IV-TR (American Psychiatric Association 2000) diagnosis of nightmare disorder is made when the patient has repeated nightmares—with the frequency and intensity impairing social, occupational, or other important functioning—and when symptoms are not attributable to another psychiatric or substance abuse disorder (see Table 5–2).

When evaluating patients with complaints of nightmares, it is important to rule out underlying medical or psychiatric illness as well as toxicity or side effects of medications, such as L-dopa, β-blockers, serotonin reuptake inhibitors, and tricyclic antidepressants. Complicated cases may merit electroencephalographic evaluation to rule out nocturnal complex partial seizures (Laberge et al. 2000).

Most patients who have nightmares have no documented psychiatric illness. Although many individuals claim an increase in nightmares secondary to stress, one study found no correlation between anxiety level and nightmare frequency. Typical treatment may include reassurance that the problem is benign, adjustment of the medication regimen, or cognitive therapy with imagery rehearsal and desensitization in milder cases.

When treating nightmares accompanying depression, anxiety disorder, or PTSD, the clinician should first emphasize treatment of underlying disorders. He or she may attempt to suppress persistent troubling nightmares with low doses of REM sleep–suppressing drugs such as antihistamines (e.g., cyproheptadine, 4–24 mg at bedtime), tricyclic antidepressants (e.g., imipramine, 10–50 mg), sedative selective serotonin reuptake inhibitors (e.g., sertraline, 50–100 mg at bedtime), mood stabilizers (e.g., carbamazepine, 100–400 mg at bedtime), or anxiolytics (e.g., clonazepam, 0.25–1.0 mg at bedtime).

TABLE 5–2.	**DSM-IV-TR diagnostic criteria for nightmare disorder**

A. Repeated awakenings from the major sleep period or naps with detailed recall of extended and extremely frightening dreams, usually involving threats to survival, security, or self-esteem. The awakenings generally occur during the second half of the sleep period.

B. On awakening from the frightening dreams, the person rapidly becomes oriented and alert (in contrast to the confusion and disorientation seen in Sleep Terror Disorder and some forms of epilepsy).

C. The dream experience, or the sleep disturbance resulting from the awakening, causes clinically significant distress or impairment in social, occupational, or other important areas of functioning.

D. The nightmares do not occur exclusively during the course of another mental disorder (e.g., a delirium, Posttraumatic Stress Disorder) and are not due to the direct physiological effects of a substance (e.g., a drug of abuse, a medication) or a general medical condition.

Sleep Paralysis

Sleep paralysis is a transient period of awakening from sleep during which the subject is unable to move or speak. Many subjects describe a sensation of weight over the chest, terror, and anxiety and feel compelled to try to move, get up, or shout. Nevertheless, in one study, 20%–25% felt calm and ignored the attacks (Wing et al. 1994).

Auditory or visual hallucinatory phenomena may accompany the paralysis, which can create a startling effect in the context of full awareness of surroundings. These would be categorized as *hypnagogic* or *hypnopompic hallucinatory phenomena,* which, like the paralysis itself, are probably related to a transition from a REM state or an admixture of REM and waking physiology.

Sleep paralysis appears to occur in three distinct groups: 1) patients with narcolepsy, who experience it as part of the narcoleptic tetrad of excessive sleepiness, cataplexy, hypnagogic hallucinations, and sleep paralysis; 2) patients with a familial type of sleep paralysis, which includes moderate daytime sleepiness, no cataplexy, and no linkage to HLADQB1*0602/DQA1*0102; and 3) people without other sleep disorders, who experience paralysis as an isolated symptom (often accompanied by hypnagogic hallucinations). Prevalence rates have been estimated from 5% to 62% in various populations, including white, black, Japanese, and Chinese people. Onset is usually in the teens, and episodes are rare after the mid-20s. Fewer than 5% of college-age students experience sleep paralysis more than once per month. The episodes appear to be triggered at times by tiredness, stress, or sleep deprivation and may often occur during naps. Sleep paralysis has also been reported as a possible side effect of antidepressant medication.

Sleep paralysis is generally treated with explanation and reassurance that it is not a dangerous phenomenon. If the paralysis is triggered by a medication, then an alternative drug could be tried. In patients who are very distraught by the experience, a REM sleep–suppressing medication (e.g., desipramine or imipramine, 10–50 mg at bedtime; or a serotonin reuptake inhibitor) may be beneficial.

The prevalence of hypnagogic and hypnopompic hallucinations is similar to that of the related phenomenon, sleep paralysis. These hallucinations also can appear as a part of the narcoleptic tetrad or as an isolated phenomenon. Treatment should be the same as that for sleep paralysis.

REM Sleep Behavior Disorder

Presenting Complaints

- Bouts of active movement during sleep
- Arm movements resulting in hitting of a bed partner
- Jumping from bed and injuring self

Clinical Presentation

REM sleep behavior disorder is a parasomnia characterized by the emergence of complex and vigorous motor behaviors during REM sleep. Punching, kicking, and leaping from the bed in an apparent attempt to enact dreams are typically seen and can cause serious physical injury. The syndrome has been described predominantly in men (90% men, 10% women) age 50 years and older (Ferini-Strambi and Zucconi 2000; Schenck and Mahowald 1996).

Etiology and Pathophysiology

The syndrome may result from damage to the brain systems controlling the normal muscle atonia of REM sleep, coupled with an enhancement of phasic motor drive. Dopaminergic mechanisms have been implicated (Albin et al. 2000). Approximately 60% of REM sleep behavior disorder cases are idiopathic. A number of cases have been associated with neurological conditions such as dementia, stroke, Parkinson's disease, multiple sclerosis, brain stem neoplasm, or atrophy. As many as 15% of patients with Parkinson's disease have REM sleep behavior disorder, and it is often present before the diagnosis of Parkinson's disease. REM sleep behavior disorder can also occur on a transient basis, secondary to toxic or metabolic conditions such as alcohol withdrawal. REM sleep behavior disorder may be associated with specific HLA antigens, with greater frequency at DQ compared with a control group.

Laboratory Findings and Diagnosis

REM sleep behavior disorder is polysomnographically characterized by one of the following patterns during REM sleep:

- Excessive augmentation of chin electromyogram (EMG) tone
- Excessive chin or limb phasic EMG twitching, irrespective of chin EMG activity, associated with abnormal behavior. This can be characterized by excessive limb or body jerking or by complex rigorous or violent movements.

There also may be increased REM density, increased slow-wave sleep, and, characteristically, an increase in limb muscle electromyographic activity in non-REM sleep, sometimes accompanied by movements.

Differential Diagnosis

The differential diagnosis includes other parasomnias, a primary sleep disorder such as apnea or periodic limb movement disorder (PLMD), gastroesophageal reflux, nocturnal seizure, PTSD, nocturnal panic disorder, and dissociative disorders. Classic polysomnographic findings are pathognomonic for REM sleep behavior disorder.

Treatment

Treatment of REM sleep behavior disorder with clonazepam has been effective in most cases. Because most patients with this disorder are elderly, a conservative approach is generally used, with the clinician starting clonazepam at a dose of 0.25 mg at bedtime and gradually increasing the dose until control is effected. If excessive daytime sedation occurs or clonazepam is ineffective, the clinician may consider REM sleep–suppressing agents with serotonergic or dopaminergic effects, such as desipramine, doxepin, carbidopa/levodopa, or clonidine, in low to intermediate doses (Mahowald and Schenck 1994).

Sleep-Related Impaired Penile Erections

Sleep-related impaired penile erections are usually detected during a laboratory study of nocturnal penile tumescence, which is most often done in the evaluation of male impotence. Laboratory evidence of impaired penile erections is usually an indication of an underlying organic factor. Major depression can impair erectile patterns during sleep, but in the context of disturbed sleep architecture. Therefore, depression should be screened for when evaluating impotence. Among the organic factors known to cause both impaired nocturnal penile tumescence and impotence are diabetes mellitus, endocrine disorders, hyperprolactinemia, penile diseases (including priapism and Peyronie's disease), central and autonomic nervous system disorders, respiratory and hematological disorders, polycythemia, lymphoma, alcoholism, psychotropic and adrenergic blocking drugs, penile arterial insufficiency, and penile venous pathology. Diagnosis requires a full medical evaluation, and treatment is directed toward correcting the underlying cause of the impaired penile erections.

Sleep-Related Painful Penile Erections

Sleep-related painful penile erections are a rare disorder in which the patient awakens several times during the night with very painful erections. After the patient awakens, the erection may slowly disappear over minutes, along with the associated pain. Although waking sexual function is usually unimpaired, serious cases result in insomnia. The clinician should evaluate the patient for underlying penile dysfunction, such as phimosis or Peyronie's disease, and start appropriate treatment. This parasomnia often does not require treatment, but in severe cases the associated insomnia may be treated with an REM sleep–suppressant drug or a sedative-hypnotic.

REM Sleep–Related Sinus Arrest

REM sleep–related sinus arrest is a rare condition that has been reported in individuals without any other apparent cardiac abnormalities and with only vague cardiac-related symptoms. These patients may experience prolonged periods of asystole, up to 9 seconds in duration, primarily during REM sleep. Patients with this condition require close cardiac follow-up and consideration for possible pacemaker implantation.

■ SLEEPWALKING AND SLEEP TERRORS

Presenting Complaints

- Nocturnal walking or confusional episodes while still apparently asleep (sleepwalking)
- Sitting up in bed, crying or screaming inconsolably, with fast heart rate and rapid breathing (sleep terrors)

- Unusual or bizarre nocturnal behavioral episodes (sleepwalking and sleep terrors)
- Initial complaints often from a parent or bed partner, because the subject usually does not recall the events (sleepwalking and sleep terrors)

Clinical Presentation

Sleepwalking, sleep terrors, and confusional arousal are related parasomnias that occur more often in children than in adults. They are characterized by motor or autonomic activity during a state of partial arousal from sleep, which is sometimes called *half-sleep* (Crisp 1996). Most children who sleepwalk do not even leave the bed; they make repetitive movements while sitting up in or on the edge of the bed. When they do leave the bed, they tend to walk around the house with their eyes open and avoid bumping into familiar objects. Their behavior tends to be quite simple in nature, and talking is minimal. Vocalization during more disturbed episodes may include crying for help, yelling about trying to escape, and possibly shouting out someone's name. When sleepwalkers are spoken to, they generally do not respond and avoid eye contact. If awakened, the sleepwalker usually experiences a period of disorientation lasting several minutes. Most sleepwalkers return to their bed in time, and one appropriate way of dealing with them is to try calmly to usher them back toward the bedroom. Attempts to awaken them are usually ineffective, may provoke physical violence, and may even prolong the episode (Laberge et al. 2000; Schenck and Mahowald 2000).

Recall of these events is usually poor or lacking, and mental content reports are more likely to have vague singular and sometimes fearful images than the typical story lines or vivid hallucinatory imagery of REM dreams. The sleepwalking episodes can last anywhere from a few seconds to a few minutes; the average episode length is about 6 minutes. Episodes up to 1 hour in duration have been reported. Sleepwalking and sleep terror episodes can be quite dangerous; approximately 75% of all patients with sleepwalking and sleep terror disorders have reported actual injuries or the potential for injuries during their episodes (Crisp 1996). One study found that more than 50% of all sleepwalkers have reported leaving the house during an episode at one time or another. Some sleepwalkers can be quite combative on sudden awakening. Some studies have found that 28%–41% of sleepwalkers and 55% of those with night terrors have reported violent behavior during these arousal episodes.

Sleep terrors are disorders of arousal that occur during the first 3 hours of the night, when Stage III and Stage IV sleep predominate. These episodes tend to begin with a loud cry and the onset of a prolonged period of apparent intense anxiety, with evidence of tachycardia, increased blood pressure, dilated pupils, and sweating. The typical episode lasts about 6 minutes. Attempts to arouse someone during a sleep terror are probably ill-advised, because disorientation may continue for up to 30 minutes after arousal from the episode (Schenck and Mahowald 2000). The episodes are more common in deep sleepers and in males and are typically not remembered the next morning (in marked contrast to nightmares during REM sleep). Persons who have sleep terrors usually calm down quickly after the episode and return to sleep.

A variation of sleep terrors that is most prevalent in children younger than 5 years is *confusional arousal*. It begins with movement and vocalization (usually crying out to parents) and often includes violent thrashing about in the bed. The child may cry uncontrollably, engage in bizarre talk, and not respond appropriately to stimulation. The parents' fear is intensified by the child's inability to be consoled, lack of response, and failure to recognize the parents, so that efforts to hold the child are ineffective or worsen the episode.

Although sleepwalking and night terror activity can appear distinctly different, elements of both often occur together in the same arousal episode. One study found that 55% of adult sleepwalkers also have sleep terrors, and 72% of persons with sleep terrors also complain of sleepwalking (Crisp 1996). Investigators have postulated that these parasomnias represent the same disorder of arousal along a continuum of severity—sleepwalking is the milder form, confusional arousal is an intermediate presentation, and sleep terrors are the most severe form of arousal.

Incidence

Of all children ages 5–12 years, 15%–40% are estimated to sleepwalk at least once, and 3%–6% sleepwalk more than once (Rosen et al. 1995). Child somnambulists usually grow out of the condition by adolescence. Surveys have estimated that 0.5%–2.5% of adults sleepwalk. Sleepwalking is highly hereditary. If both parents sleepwalk, there is a 60% chance that any of their children will sleepwalk (Crisp 1996; Schenck and Mahowald 2000). If only one parent sleepwalks, the risk is reduced to 45%. Among all age groups, the incidence of sleep terrors appears to be significantly less than that of sleepwalking, and the incidence of sleep terrors is probably about 1%–2% among children (Rosen et al. 1995).

Etiology and Pathophysiology

Sleepwalking and sleep terrors are disorders of arousal usually from slow-wave or Stage III and Stage IV non-REM sleep, which may reflect an impairment (developmental or other) in the normal mechanisms of arousal from deep sleep. This impairment results in partial arousals, during which motor behaviors are activated but full consciousness is not restored. This may be one reason that parasomnias are more common in the "immature" nervous system of children and that children typically grow out of them.

Discerning the etiology of nocturnal partial arousals requires sorting out environmental and genetic components as well as predisposing and precipitating factors. Although the hereditary nature of sleepwalking and sleep terrors is clear, the degree of genetic loading can vary significantly. In some patients, specific stressors or traumas may be necessary to elicit the symptoms, whereas in patients with a very strong genetic loading, sleepwalking and night terrors may persist into adulthood without evidence of stress, trauma, or psychological disturbance.

Predisposing factors for nocturnal partial arousals are sleep deprivation (very important), chaotic sleep–wake schedules, emotional trauma and loss, psychotic illness, and migraine headaches. Precipitating factors for sleepwalking include obstructive sleep apnea, seizures, fever, PLMD, alcohol, stress, and gastroesophageal reflux. Other precipitants include turning on lights, touching the patient, and treatment with certain medications, including cardiac drugs such as propranolol, antiarrhythmics, neuroleptics, diazepam, and sedatives.

Laboratory Findings

Nocturnal polysomnographic recordings during somnambulistic or sleep terror episodes most commonly show an arousal from Stage III sleep or Stage IV non-REM sleep; however, at times, these episodes may occur during any non-REM sleep state. The behavioral disturbance is often preceded by generalized, hypersynchronous, symmetric, high-amplitude delta patterns on the electroencephalogram (EEG). Heart rate and breathing increase at onset of the partial arousal. The electroencephalographic findings are quite different from those in REM sleep behavior disorder, which emerges from a typical REM state with a low-voltage, fast EEG.

Differential Diagnosis

Nightmares tend to occur during REM sleep in the middle of the night or in the morning. Because REM sleep induces muscle paralysis, nightmares are not associated with movement. The person tends to have good recall of the dream afterward and becomes alert and calm soon after awakening.

Automatic behavior and *dissociative states* are usually found in adults with psychiatric disturbances. Often such events occur during waking and sleep states. Behavior may be much more complex than that seen in a typical sleepwalking or sleep terror episode. Episodes involving automatic behavior and dissociative states can last several hours, and the person frequently does not return to his or her own bed.

Sleep drunkenness is a state of partial awakening that results when an individual is extremely fatigued or affected by sedatives or alcohol. This state may also be seen as part of the narcolepsy syndrome. Although aggressive behavior is common during this state, there is no good evidence that a patient can intentionally commit a criminal act during such episodes without having some awareness.

Psychomotor epileptic seizures tend to be short, and no response can be elicited from the patient during the episodes. An EEG may be necessary to distinguish these episodes from sleepwalking or sleep terrors. The EEG should be done after a night of partial sleep deprivation and should include an adequate sleep recording.

Panic attacks may be confused with parasomnias. It is common for patients with nocturnal panic attacks to present with episodes of tachycardia, shortness of breath, sweating, and extreme fear or terror. The main distinction between the panic attack and sleep terrors is that the patient is alert and aware of surroundings during the panic attack and has very clear recall of the onset and the events surrounding the episode the next morning.

REM sleep behavior disorder may be confused with sleep terrors. However, the sudden onset in elderly patients that is characteristic of REM sleep behavior disorder is not characteristic of sleep terrors. Polysomnographic findings can clearly differentiate the two disorders.

Sleep apnea or *periodic leg movements* trigger arousal. Polysomnographic findings can distinguish these syndromes from sleepwalking and sleep terrors.

A toxic reaction to drugs, a brain injury, or *dementia with episodic nocturnal wandering* also must be differentiated from sleepwalking and sleep terrors.

Specific laboratory studies are usually unnecessary for the diagnosis of sleepwalking and sleep terrors. DSM-IV-TR diagnostic criteria for sleepwalking disorder and sleep terror disorder are shown in Tables 5–3 and 5–4, respectively. In persistent cases of these disorders, especially those in which the clinician may have some concern about possible psychomotor epilepsy, an EEG may be indicated. If confusion or concern about persistent and frequent

TABLE 5–3. **DSM-IV-TR diagnostic criteria for sleepwalking disorder**

A. Repeated episodes of rising from bed during sleep and walking about, usually occurring during the first third of the major sleep episode.

B. While sleepwalking, the person has a blank, staring face, is relatively unresponsive to the efforts of others to communicate with him or her, and can be awakened only with great difficulty.

C. On awakening (either from the sleepwalking episode or the next morning), the person has amnesia for the episode.

D. Within several minutes after awakening from the sleepwalking episode, there is no impairment of mental activity or behavior (although there may initially be a short period of confusion or disorientation).

E. The sleepwalking causes clinically significant distress or impairment in social, occupational, or other important areas of functioning.

F. The disturbance is not due to the direct physiological effects of a substance (e.g., a drug of abuse, a medication) or a general medical condition.

TABLE 5–4. **DSM-IV-TR diagnostic criteria for sleep terror disorder**

A. Recurrent episodes of abrupt awakening from sleep, usually occurring during the first third of the major sleep episode and beginning with a panicky scream.

B. Intense fear and signs of autonomic arousal, such as tachycardia, rapid breathing, and sweating, during each episode.

C. Relative unresponsiveness to efforts of others to comfort the person during the episode.

D. No detailed dream is recalled and there is amnesia for the episode.

E. The episodes cause clinically significant distress or impairment in social, occupational, or other important areas of functioning.

F. The disturbance is not due to the direct physiological effects of a substance (e.g., a drug of abuse, a medication) or a general medical condition.

problems remains, a polysomnogram (PSG) could be obtained to clarify whether the episodes indeed are occurring early in the night during Stage III or Stage IV sleep and to rule out REM sleep behavior disorder. The PSG could also provide information regarding whether electroencephalographic abnormalities are present during nocturnal sleep but not seen on a routine EEG. Videotaping the patient during polysomnographic recording, to correlate behavior and recording, is important.

Treatment

Treatment is dependent on the type of clinical presentation. Most children with somnambulism or sleep terrors grow out of the symptoms as they physiologically mature. The clinician should reassure the parents and the child. Sleepwalkers should be protected by appropriate locks on the doors and windows to preclude the patient's leaving the house and being put in a dangerous position. Hazardous objects should also be removed, and windows should be covered with heavy drapes. Inexpensive ultrasonic burglar alarms can be used to alert others in the house that the patient has started walking. The sleepwalker should sleep on the first floor to avoid the risk of falling out of a window. The patient must avoid sleep deprivation and exercise good sleep hygiene. In severe cases, a therapist should explore the possibility of psychotherapy, behavior therapy, or hypnosis. Behavior therapies should focus on relaxation and soothing mental imagery.

When sleepwalking episodes are frequent and predictable, anticipatory awakening for 5 minutes about 30 minutes before the event usually begins has been shown to be effective on occasion (Tobin 1993). Treatment-resistant patients may require a low dose of a tricyclic (e.g., imipramine, 10–50 mg) or a benzodiazepine (e.g., triazolam, 0.125 mg; or diazepam, 2 mg at bedtime), which may decrease the frequency of the events either by suppressing arousal or by suppressing deep Stage III and Stage IV sleep.

Sleepwalking and sleep terrors in adults are frequently amenable to psychotherapeutic intervention, progressive relaxation, or hypnosis. At our center, a number of patients have been treated with short-term exploratory and insight-oriented therapy, including helping the patient to express emotions more directly. Sleepwalking and sleep terror symptoms were alleviated within a matter of weeks. For those who have potentially dangerous sleepwalking and sleep terror episodes, medication is the most appropriate treatment to consider early on, in conjunction with psychotherapy. At our center, clinicians frequently begin treatment with desipramine (10 mg at bedtime) and gradually increase the dose until the episodes diminish significantly. Imipramine, nortriptyline, sertraline, paroxetine, carbamazepine, diazepam, triazolam, and divalproex have also been used successfully. Although most patients respond to relatively low doses of these drugs, patients who have evidence of concurrent depression require full antidepressant doses. The same protective measures just recommended for children should be instituted for adults as well.

In elderly patients, new-onset sleepwalking is often a result of medication side effects, possibly combined with underlying medical illness. If medication is prescribed, the clinician must be careful not to aggravate a preexisting confusional state.

■ SLEEP–WAKE TRANSITION DISORDERS

Sleep–wake transition disorders tend to occur during the transition from wakefulness to sleep or sleep to wakefulness and represent altered physiological processes rather than true pathological changes.

Sleep starts include hypnic jerks and sensory starts. A *hypnic jerk* is a generalized body jerk that occurs at the onset of sleep. Hypnic jerks are almost universal, nonpathological, and probably a minor arousal response to some subtle stimulus at the time of sleep onset. *Sensory starts* include sensory experiences, often of a dreamlike nature, that can accompany a hypnic jerk or occur by themselves at the time of sleep onset and can bring one back into wakefulness. Sensory starts are benign. The clinician should treat both forms of sleep starts by reassuring the patient that these conditions are normal.

Sleeptalking is a very common event that most often occurs during the transition to Stage I or Stage II sleep. It often occurs when an individual who is just falling asleep is asked a question. The patient often does not recall what he or she has said. Extreme tiredness may make sleeptalking more likely. Sleeptalking does not seem to be closely associated with other arousal disorders such as sleepwalking or sleep terrors. Sleeptalking is seldom of any medical concern on its own and is generally nonresponsive to medication or psychotherapy.

■ OTHER PARASOMNIAS

Nocturnal Sleep–Related Eating Disorder

Presenting Complaints

- Repeated arousals from sleep that are associated with overeating, often with partial or no awareness before morning
- Overeating behavior that often occurs nightly or is out of control and resistant to intervention by the overeater or others

Clinical Presentation

Some patients awaken frequently and recurrently to eat or drink (Schenck et al. 1993; Winkleman 1998). Degrees of awareness of the eating behavior vary. In many subjects, the overeating behavior can occur nightly and usually involves an immediate and compulsive urge to eat high-calorie foods (e.g., sweets or carbohydrates) despite a lack of awareness of real hunger or thirst. The excessive intake may cause weight gain and abdominal distension. This eating disorder is not usually accompanied by purging or daytime binge eating. Onset may be related to stressful life events or physical illness, and associated depressive disorders are common. Comorbid psychiatric illness is common, but patients tend to function well.

Incidence

Nocturnal sleep–related eating disorder is most likely a rare syndrome, but embarrassment, self-blame, and failure to respond to various interventions may contribute to its being underreported.

Etiology and Pathophysiology

Nocturnal sleep–related eating disorder may have multiple and complex predispositions and causes, including a family history of parasomnia; may occur with other sleep disorders (e.g., obstructive sleep apnea, PLMD, restless legs syndrome); and may be related to current stress or early abuse. Many patients have concurrent depression. Researchers have postulated that nocturnal sleep–related eating may be associated with low central nervous system dopamine and serotonin activity.

Laboratory Findings

Nocturnal polysomnographic data from this group suggest an atypical form of adult sleepwalking in some and atypical awakenings in others. There appear to be abrupt arousals from non-REM sleep at the onset of the episodes of sleep-related eating. The incidence of obstructive sleep apnea, PLMD, and restless legs syndrome may be increased.

Differential Diagnosis

Nocturnal sleep–related eating is distinguished from other disorders by the minimal or total lack of consciousness of the eating behavior. Patients with bulimia tend to engage in daytime bingeing as well. Anxiety disorders and atypical depression may have hyperphagia components triggered chemically or in response to a need for self-soothing behavior.

Treatment

The clinician should evaluate the patient for mood and anxiety disorders or substance abuse and should treat these disorders appropriately. If bipolar disorder is present or suspected, use of a mood stabilizer such as carbamazepine or valproic acid may be appropriate as an initial treatment. Other patients with mood, anxiety, or substance use disorders may benefit from a trial of fluoxetine (20–60 mg) or an alternative serotonin reuptake inhibitor. A dopamine agonist such as carbidopa/levodopa (10/100 mg; up to three tablets at bedtime), bromocriptine (2.5–15 mg), or pergolide (0.05–0.5 mg) might be considered. If these medications are ineffective, propoxyphene or 30 mg of codeine (one to three tablets of either at bedtime) should be added to the dopamine agonist. Patients who still do not respond may benefit from the addition of clonazepam (0.25–2.0 mg at bedtime). Milder cases may respond to clonazepam alone, and more complicated cases may require all the listed medications.

The clinician should not neglect adjunctive treatments such as practicing sleep hygiene, reducing stress, undergoing individual or relationship therapy if indicated, and eliminating unnecessary drugs or medications.

Sleep Bruxism

Sleep bruxism is a very common disorder consisting of repetitive, sometimes violent, teeth grinding during sleep. Bruxism has a reported prevalence ranging from 7% to 88% in children and decreases in frequency with age. Bruxism probably has no single etiology, but causative factors include genetics, anatomical disturbance (jaw malformation or malocclusion), central nervous system dysfunction (comatose and developmentally disabled patients are at increased risk), and psychological disorders (exacerbated by anxiety and stress). Also, cases of bruxism have been reported secondary to orofacial dyskinesia, mandibular dystonia, tremors, and REM sleep behavior disorders. Bruxism occurs mainly during Stage II sleep. On the PSG, increased amplitude of electromyographic activity in the masseter and the temporalis muscles is evident. A formal sleep study may be necessary to rule out nocturnal seizures. The treatment of choice is a dental device to avoid damaging and wearing down the teeth. Other treatments that have had occasional success include muscle relaxation exercises, hypnotic medication, biofeedback, hypnosis, occlusal adjustment, corrective dental surgery, and psychotherapy. Other newer treatments that show promise include botulinum toxin injection for those with orofacial dystonia and dyskinesia and contingent afferent stimulation of the lip for patients with uncomplicated bruxism.

Benign Neonatal Sleep Myoclonus

Benign neonatal sleep myoclonus is a rare syndrome of rhythmic jerking of hands, arms, and legs, as well as occasional repetitive jerking of fingers, wrists, elbows, and ankles, that occurs in early infancy. The movements may occur at sleep onset as well as later in sleep. Symptoms tend to disappear by ages 1–2 years. This benign condition can be diagnosed by the presence of normal electroencephalographic findings and by the fact that it occurs only during sleep. The syndrome is thought to represent a developmental abnormality in the reticular activating system, possibly related to sleep starts, that resolves with maturation of the nervous system.

Nocturnal Dissociative Disorders

Nocturnal dissociative disorders involve elaborate behaviors that appear to represent attempts to reenact abusive situations from earlier in life, especially childhood or adolescent sexual abuse. The episodes tend to arise during periods of wakefulness occurring after episodes of sleep. A patient with a nocturnal dissociative disorder should be treated with psychotherapy and pharmacotherapy directed toward the dissociative disorder and accompanying psychiatric disorders. Nocturnal dissociative disorders may be aggravated by bedtime administration of benzodiazepines.

Nocturnal Muscle Cramps

Nocturnal muscle cramps are occasionally familial and subjectively shown to respond to quinine sulfate or verapamil.

Central Nervous System Parasomnias

Nocturnal paroxysmal dystonia is a rare syndrome of often violent movements of the limbs and trunk that occur during non-REM sleep. No associated abnormalities are revealed by standard electroencephalography, magnetic resonance imaging, computed tomography, or neurological examination. Patients tend to fall asleep after the episodes. They maintain at least partial recall of the events if awakened and questioned. Episodes tend to occur nightly and may occur as often as 20 times per night. They are categorized according to their duration. Ultrashort episodes (8–20 seconds) are termed *paroxysmal arousal,* and dystonic episodes less than 2 minutes are called *nocturnal paroxysmal dystonia with short-lasting attacks.* Intermediate-duration or long attacks (2–50 minutes) tend to be much less responsive to treatment. If this disorder is suspected, the clinician should still evaluate the patient with a neurological examination, electroencephalography, computed tomography, or magnetic resonance imaging and videotape-monitored nocturnal polysomnography to rule out other neurological disorders or parasomnias. The PSG in nocturnal paroxysmal dystonia will show an arousal at the beginning of the episode but seldom any electroencephalographic findings suggestive of epilepsy. Some data suggest that patients with nocturnal paroxysmal dystonia have an epileptic focus on the frontal lobe; thus, this abnormality may represent a nocturnal seizure disorder (Montagna 1992).

The short episodes respond well to carbamazepine. Treatment should begin with carbamazepine (200 mg at bedtime), and the dose should be increased until the patient responds to the treatment or toxicity develops. If the patient does not respond to carbamazepine, the clinician should try phenytoin (5 mg/kg in two to three divided doses), barbiturates (e.g., phenobarbital, 100–150 mg at bedtime), or other anticonvulsants. No treatments have yet been shown to be effective for attacks lasting longer than 2 minutes.

Vascular headaches include cluster headaches, chronic paroxysmal hemicrania, and migraines and are in some cases REM sleep related. Often symptoms worsen as a part of REM rebound after discontinuation of REM sleep–suppressing agents such as antidepressants. Episodic paroxysmal hemicrania may respond to calcium-channel blockers. Obstructive sleep apnea can trigger cluster headaches.

Exploding head syndrome is usually a benign syndrome of abrupt arousal occurring in the early transition into sleep, with a complaint of a sensation of a loud sound like an explosion or a sensation of bursting in the head. This syndrome is most likely a variant of hypnic jerks, although a seizure disorder may need to be ruled out in persistent or complicated cases. A related condition, hypnic headache syndrome, was described in a number of elderly patients as a diffuse headache awakening the patient from a dream, lasting 30–60 minutes, and accompanied by nausea (Mahowald and Schenck 1996). Symptoms improve with administration of lithium.

Cardiopulmonary Parasomnias

Respiratory dyskinesias include segmental myoclonus, palatal myoclonus, diaphragmatic flutter, and paroxysmal dystonia. They may be manifestations of neuroleptic-induced dyskinesias. They should be differentiated from nocturnal seizures with primarily respiratory symptoms.

Sudden unexplained nocturnal death syndrome is a syndrome of unexpected nocturnal death occurring in young Asian males. The syndrome is known as *bangungut* in the Philippines, *nonlaitai* in Laos, and *pokkuri* in Japan (Melles and Katz 1988). Cardiac conduction defects have been found in postmortem analysis in many of the victims, and there is evidence that many victims also had sleep terrors. These findings suggest a relationship between the autonomic arousal associated with sleep terrors and the cardiac conduction abnormalities leading to nocturnal death.

Gastrointestinal Parasomnias

Gastroesophageal reflux can occur during sleep, presenting as abrupt awakenings, choking, chest pain, dyspnea, or severe anxiety. It can produce prolonged laryngospasm, cause pulmonary aspiration, or aggravate bronchial asthma. Diagnosis may require nocturnal esophageal pH monitoring. Medical treatment usually involves decreasing stomach acid with histamine-2 blockers or proton pump blockers. Elevating the head of the bed may also be beneficial.

Diffuse esophageal spasm or *nocturnal esophageal spasms* create chest pain and mimic cardiac disease, and they have been known to trigger arrhythmias. Diagnosis can be made by measuring esophageal pressure or by endoscopy. Successful treatments have included administration of calcium-channel blockers, nitrates, or anticholinergic agents.

Sleep-related tonic spasms or *proctalgia fugax* is intense spasms of the levator ani muscle that can cause excruciating pain. The pain is usually felt in the rectum just above the anus and can last from a few seconds to a half hour. There is still no known organic cause. The syndrome may have some relationship to anxiety. It occasionally occurs during the daytime as well as at night. No effective treatment is available other than reassurance that it will not progress or lead to more serious problems.

Sleep-related abnormal swallowing syndrome is characterized by complaints of choking on pooled saliva that has not been swallowed during sleep. No clear treatment is available for the disorder, but patients should be evaluated for the presence of a pharyngeal pouch.

■ AGGRESSIVE AND VIOLENT BEHAVIOR DURING SLEEP

Aggressive and violent behaviors can accompany sleep disorders. REM sleep behavior disorder can result in violence as patients act out dream content, with potential injury to both patient and bed partner (Ohayon et al. 1997). Patients have committed homicide during somnambulistic episodes, and parasomnias have become a legal defense on occasion. A well-known case is that of Kenneth Parks, a 23-year-old man who stabbed his mother-in-law to death as part of a somnambulistic episode. He was found not guilty of murder, because murder requires intent, and his somnambulistic episode was considered to be a noninsane automatism, without intent (Broughton et al. 1994).

Individuals with violent behavior during sleep have also been shown to have higher incidences of sleep talking, bruxism, hypnic jerks, hypnagogic hallucinations, and anxiety and mood disorders, as well as increased levels of smoking, caffeine use, and bedtime alcohol ingestion. A thorough workup is required for accurate assessment of violence resulting in criminal charges during sleep. A comprehensive discussion of this topic is beyond the scope of this volume, but several publications include in-depth descriptions of this subject (Broughton and Shimizu 1995; Mahowald and Schenck 1995).

■ REFERENCES

Albin RL, Koeppe RA, Chervin RD, et al: Decreased striatal dopaminergic innervation in REM sleep behavior disorder. Neurology 55:1410–1412, 2000

American Psychiatric Association: Diagnostic and Statistical Manual of Mental Disorders, 4th Edition, Text Revision (DSM-IV-TR). Washington, DC, American Psychiatric Association, 2000

Broughton R, Shimizu T: Sleep-related violence: a medical and forensic challenge. Sleep 18:727–730, 1995

Broughton R, Billings R, Cartwright D, et al: Homicidal somnambulism: a case report. Sleep 17:253–264, 1994

Crisp AH: The sleepwalking/night terrors syndrome in adults. Postgrad Med J 72:599–604, 1996

Ferini-Strambi L, Zucconi M: REM sleep behavior disorder. Clin Neurophysiol 111(suppl 2):S136–S140, 2000

Laberge L, Tremblay R, Vitaro F, et al: Development of parasomnias from childhood to early adolescence. Pediatrics 106:67–74, 2000

Mahowald MW, Schenck CH: REM sleep behavior disorder, in Principles and Practice of Sleep Medicine. Edited by Kryger MH, Roth T, Dement WC. Philadelphia, PA, WB Saunders, 1994, pp 574–588

Mahowald MW, Schenck CH: Complex motor behavior arising during the sleep period: forensic science implications. Sleep 18:724–727, 1995

Mahowald MW, Schenck CH: NREM sleep parasomnias. Neurol Clin 14:675–696, 1996

Melles RB, Katz B: Night terrors and sudden unexplained nocturnal death. Med Hypotheses 26:149–154, 1988

Montagna P: Nocturnal paroxysmal dystonia and nocturnal wandering. Neurology 42:61–67, 1992

Ohayon M, Caulet M, Priest R: Violent behavior during sleep. J Clin Psychiatry 58:369–376, 1997

Rosen G, Mahowald MW, Ferber R: Sleepwalking, confusional arousals, and sleep terrors in the child, in Principles and Practice of Sleep Medicine in the Child. Edited by Ferber R, Kryger M. Philadelphia, PA, WB Saunders, 1995, pp 99–106

Ross RJ, Ball WA, Dinges DF, et al: Motor dysfunction during sleep in posttraumatic stress disorder. Sleep 17:723–732, 1994

Schenck CH, Mahowald MW: REM sleep parasomnias. Neurol Clin 14:697–720, 1996

Schenck CH, Mahowald MW: Parasomnias. Managing bizarre sleep-related behavior disorders. Postgrad Med 107:145–156, 2000

Schenck CH, Hurwitz TD, O'Connor KA, et al: Additional categories of sleep-related eating disorders and the current status of treatment. Sleep 16:457–466, 1993

Tobin JD: Treatment of somnambulism with anticipatory awakening. J Pediatr 122:426–427, 1993

Wing Y-K, Lee ST, Chen C-N: Sleep paralysis in Chinese: ghost oppression phenomenon in Hong Kong. Sleep 17:609–613, 1994

Winkleman JW: Clinical and polysomnographic features of sleep-related eating disorder. J Clin Psychiatry 59:14–19, 1998

6

MEDICAL AND PSYCHIATRIC DISORDERS AND SLEEP

Sleep can be disrupted by *symptoms* associated with medical illnesses (e.g., insomnia due to arthritic pain), by the *medical condition* itself (e.g., hypersomnia due to neoplasms of the central nervous system [CNS]), or by *drugs* used to treat the medical condition. In most cases, the sleep complaint tends to wax and wane along with the medical illness. If the sleep abnormality persists after the underlying medical condition improves, other factors (e.g., psychophysiological or conditioned insomnia) may have become involved.

■ SYMPTOMS OF MEDICAL DISORDERS DISRUPTIVE TO SLEEP

Frequent symptoms that may accompany a large variety of medical disorders and that may significantly disrupt sleep include abnormal movements from any cause, diarrhea, night sweats, nocturia, nocturnal confusion, pain from any cause, palpitations, pruritus, and respiratory symptoms.

■ SPECIFIC MEDICAL CONDITIONS ASSOCIATED WITH DISORDERED SLEEP

When the direct physiological effects of a medical condition cause a sleep disturbance, the DSM-IV-TR (American Psychiatric Association 2000) diagnosis is sleep disorder due to a general medical condition (see Table 6–1).

TABLE 6–1. **DSM-IV-TR diagnostic criteria for sleep disorder due to a general medical condition**

A. A prominent disturbance in sleep that is sufficiently severe to warrant independent clinical attention.

B. There is evidence from the history, physical examination, or laboratory findings that the sleep disturbance is the direct physiological consequence of a general medical condition.

C. The disturbance is not better accounted for by another mental disorder (e.g., an Adjustment Disorder in which the stressor is a serious medical illness).

D. The disturbance does not occur exclusively during the course of a delirium.

E. The disturbance does not meet the criteria for Breathing-Related Sleep Disorder or Narcolepsy.

F. The sleep disturbance causes clinically significant distress or impairment in social, occupational, or other important areas of functioning.

Specify type:

   Insomnia Type: if the predominant sleep disturbance is insomnia
   Hypersomnia Type: if the predominant sleep disturbance is hypersomnia
   Parasomnia Type: if the predominant sleep disturbance is a Parasomnia
   Mixed Type: if more than one sleep disturbance is present and none predominates

Coding note: Include the name of the general medical condition on Axis I, e.g., 780.52 Sleep Disorder Due to Chronic Obstructive Pulmonary Disease, Insomnia Type; also code the general medical condition on Axis III.

Cardiac diseases are often associated with poor sleep. Cardiac dysrhythmias, angina pectoris, and breathing disorders all can cause awakenings and sleep fragmentation. Sleep state–related changes in sympathetic and parasympathetic nervous system activity as well as changes in blood pressure may contribute to cardiac dysrhythmias and ischemia. Sympathetic activity can abruptly increase during rapid eye movement (REM) sleep (especially with phasic eye movements), leading to coronary vasoconstriction and an acceleration of heart rate. Increased parasympathetic activity can induce bradycardia and even sinus pauses. Hypotension can occur in non-REM sleep (especially slow-wave sleep) and decrease coronary artery perfusion in narrowed vessels. These sleep-related mechanisms may induce cardiac dysrhythmias and ischemia in individuals with existing cardiac vascular disease. Patients with congestive heart failure have been shown to have a high incidence of sleep-related breathing disorders (Javaheri et al. 1995)—frequently, a combination of Cheyne-Stokes respiration and central and obstructive apneas. Supplemental oxygen is commonly used in cases of Cheyne-Stokes respiration and central sleep apnea. Nasal continuous positive airway pressure (CPAP) therapy has been shown to be quite helpful in improving oxygenation, left ventricular function, respiration during sleep, and sleep quality in patients with congestive heart failure associated with either Cheyne-Stokes respiration or sleep apnea (both central and obstructive) (Naughton et al. 1994). A relative reduction in the risk of death on receiving a heart transplant has also been shown in patients treated with CPAP therapy (Sin et al. 2000).

CNS neoplasms can cause movement disorders or seizures leading to insomnia. Midline lesions (in the pineal gland, hypothalamus, third ventricle, or brain stem) often lead to increased intracranial pressure. Patients with these lesions may have increased sleepiness, ranging from mildly increased daytime somnolence to obtundation. Patients with subdural hematomas, multiple sclerosis, neurosyphilis, a seizure disorder, trypanosomiasis, or head trauma or who are postencephalitic frequently have excessive daytime sleepiness (EDS).

Degenerative diseases of the CNS often are associated with insomnia characterized by frequent awakenings and a reduced amount of Stage III, Stage IV, and REM sleep. Although the characteristic tremor of Parkinson's disease decreases during sleep, it returns during many of the frequent arousals. Diseases involving degeneration in the medulla and pons (e.g., olivopontocerebellar degeneration, progressive supranuclear palsy, and Parkinson's disease) can lead to or be preceded by REM sleep behavior disorder (see Chapter 5) and frequent limb jerks. Respiratory abnormalities (such as central and obstructive apnea) often occur in patients who have autonomic dysfunction as part of a CNS degenerative condition (e.g., Parkinson's disease or Shy-Drager syndrome). These patients may be at increased risk for sudden death during sleep (Munschauer et al. 1990). The clinician should consider early polysomnographic evaluation and assess the need for aggressive management to maintain patency of the airway (with nasal CPAP therapy or tracheostomy) during sleep. Dementing illnesses are associated with fragmented sleep (due to arousals and awakenings) and decreased sleep efficiency. Patients with severe dementia may develop a day–night reversal, often with agitation in the evening (sundowning) and night. These behaviors are a major cause of nursing home placement of elderly patients.

Fatal familial insomnia is a rare degenerative disorder that typically presents with severe insomnia, endocrine abnormalities, dysautonomia, and degeneration of thalamic nuclei (Montagna et al. 1995). The insomnia is characterized by a decrease in both slow-wave and REM sleep. As the disease progresses, hallucinations, ataxia, myoclonus, and, later, stupor occur. Hyperthermia, tachycardia, and hypertension are aspects of the dysautonomia. This untreatable condition is believed to be an inherited prion disease, but it may occur sporadically as well.

Endocrinopathies are notorious for disrupting sleep. Patients with hypothyroidism frequently complain of fatigue and sleepiness and have a decrease in Stage III and Stage IV sleep that normalizes with thyroid hormone supplementation. Respiratory disorders such as sleep apnea and abnormal respiratory drive have been reported in patients with hypothyroidism (VanDyck et al. 1989). Infants with hypothyroidism have decreased sleep spindles, and spindles increase after hormone therapy. Patients with hyperthyroidism have increased Stage III and Stage IV sleep before treatment. Cushing's syndrome and Addison's disease have been associated with insomnia. Patients with Cushing's syndrome tend to have decreased amounts of slow-wave sleep and may be prone to develop obstructive sleep apnea. Those with Addison's disease also have decreased amounts of Stage III and Stage IV sleep.

Diabetes can lead to poor sleep for a variety of reasons. Nocturnal hypoglycemia (Somogyi effect), nocturnal diarrhea, and pain from peripheral neuropathies all can disrupt sleep.

Primary pulmonary disorders such as chronic obstructive pulmonary disease, cystic fibrosis, and asthma may be associated with significant sleep disturbance and associated complaints. These disorders are discussed in more detail in Chapter 4.

Fibromyalgia and *chronic fatigue syndrome* (CFS) are conditions in which patients complain of myalgia, arthralgia, chronic fatigue, and nonrestorative sleep. In patients with fibromyalgia, physical examination is notable for characteristic "tender points" (such as on the trapezius, the medial fat pad on the knee, the iliac crest, and the lateral epicondyle). Polysomnograms (PSGs) in these patients often show an increased amount of alpha-frequency activity throughout non-REM sleep; such sleep is sometimes referred to as *alpha-delta sleep* (see Figure 6–1). Although this alpha-delta pattern is not specific to fibromyalgia or CFS, it may represent a physiological arousal disorder perceived by the patient as nonrestorative sleep (Harding 1998). Some patients with fibromyalgia and CFS have other primary sleep disorders, such as periodic limb movement disorder (PLMD), sleep apnea, or narcolepsy, which suggests that a PSG may be an appropriate component of the evaluation (Krupp et al. 1993).

Epstein-Barr virus infection often induces sleep complaints such as insomnia and nonrestorative sleep. Studies show frequent polysomnographic abnormalities in patients with Epstein-Barr virus infection. These abnormalities are of various types, including alpha-delta patterns.

Arthritis may be associated with poor sleep, including frequent arousals and an increase in alpha-frequency activity in the sleep electroencephalogram (EEG). Some studies have suggested that patients with osteoarthritis and significant morning stiffness may have PLMD and alpha intrusion.

Chronic renal failure is associated with poor nighttime sleep, prolonged awakenings, and EDS. Restless legs syndrome is a com-

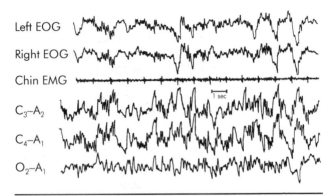

FIGURE 6–1. **Excessive alpha-frequency activity superimposed on basically delta slow-wave sleep background.**

This illustration was taken from the polysomnographic record of a 41-year-old woman with sleep complaints of both insomnia and excessive daytime sleepiness and with a possible Epstein-Barr virus infection. The patient was taking alprazolam (1 mg/day) and trazodone (150 mg/day).

A_1=left ear; A_2=right ear; C_3=left high central electroencephalogram (EEG); C_4=right high central EEG; EMG=electromyogram; EOG=electro-oculogram; O_2=right occipital EEG.

mon complaint in this group. Polysomnographic studies have found a relatively high incidence of sleep apnea and PLMD in patients with chronic renal failure. Dialysis may be related to improved sleep architecture, with increased Stage III and Stage IV sleep. Some studies indicate "cures" of sleep apnea with dialysis or renal transplantation (Fein et al. 1987; Langevin et al. 1993), whereas other studies indicate persistent sleep apnea after treatment (Mendelson et al. 1990).

Anorexia nervosa often is associated with sleep-onset and sleep-maintenance insomnia. Patients with anorexia also have early-morning awakenings. Polysomnographic recordings have demonstrated decreased total sleep time, slow-wave sleep, and REM sleep latency. Sleep tends to improve as these patients gain weight.

Gastric acid secretion during sleep is up to 20 times greater than normal in patients with peptic ulcer disease. Nocturnal pain from peptic ulcer disease, as well as nocturnal gastroesophageal reflux or regurgitation, can disrupt sleep.

Chronic headache may cause insomnia, decrease total sleep time, and result in frequent arousals. Patients with cluster or migraine headaches or chronic paroxysmal hemicrania frequently report that their headaches begin during sleep. Polysomnographic studies show that such headaches often start during, or shortly after, an episode of REM sleep.

Asymptomatic and symptomatic AIDS may result in both EDS and insomnia. Studies involving asymptomatic patients infected with HIV have shown an increase in slow-wave sleep, especially during the second part of the night, as well as a decrease in sleep efficiency. As the HIV progresses, sleep becomes more fragmented, with frequent arousals; slow-wave sleep decreases; and rhythmic REM/non-REM cycles are suppressed (Norman et al. 1992).

Many *toxic states* induced by medications or chemical exposure are associated with decreased and fragmented sleep. Carbon monoxide, mercury, arsenic, and cytotoxic chemotherapeutic agents for malignancies are a few of the compounds in this category.

Sleep disturbances can be seen as *side effects* of a substantial number of commonly used pharmacological agents (see Table 3–1 in Chapter 3). The sleep complaint begins shortly after initiation of drug therapy or after a dose increase and decreases when the medication is withdrawn. Caffeine and nicotine may also disturb sleep in such a manner.

Studies involving patients who have undergone *surgical procedures* or who are in *intensive care units* indicate that sleep in these patients is fragmented, with frequent arousals, and contains very little Stage III, Stage IV, or REM sleep. Many awakenings are caused by nursing activities such as checking vital signs or administering medication. Nurses often overestimate the amount of sleep that patients actually obtain.

■ TREATMENT OF SLEEP COMPLAINTS IN PATIENTS WITH MEDICAL ILLNESS

The proper treatment of any patient with disordered sleep begins with the correct diagnosis. The clinician must consider the effect of the primary medical illness on sleep, the consequences of therapies for the medical problem, and the possibility of coexisting primary sleep disorders.

If the sleep complaint is believed to be related directly to an underlying medical problem, the initial effort should be to improve that primary condition as well as those symptoms disruptive to sleep. If the sleep complaint persists or worsens after the medical problem is controlled, the clinician must determine whether aspects of the treatment modalities themselves may be contributing to the problem.

If the sleep complaint persists after resolution of the medical illness, a primary sleep disorder likely exists. Persistent psychophysiological insomnia (conditional arousal) commonly arises as a result of an acute medical illness. The clinician also must consider the presence of unsuspected primary sleep disorders such as PLMD or sleep apnea. In some patients, a polysomnographic evaluation is necessary to make the correct diagnosis.

Patients who are thought to have fibrositis often respond to small doses of amitriptyline (10–50 mg/day) or cyclobenzaprine (10 mg three times a day). Nonsteroidal anti-inflammatory drugs occasionally are beneficial. In patients with fibrositis, a PSG may be very useful in evaluating possible concurrent PLMD. If PLMD is found, the clinician should consider use of a benzodiazepine hypnotic, such as temazepam or clonazepam, and should avoid administering tricyclic antidepressants.

Patients who have insomnia associated with an acute medical illness and who have no other contraindication may be treated for a short time with hypnotics. Ideally, medications with a short half-life, such as zolpidem (5–10 mg at bedtime), zaleplon (5–20 mg), or triazolam (0.125–0.25 mg at bedtime), should be used.

The summary guidelines provided in Table 6–2 may be helpful for treatment of insomnia in patients with medical illness.

TABLE 6–2.	Guidelines for treatment of insomnia in patients with medical illness

1. Make a diagnosis.
2. Treat the medical illness first.
3. Determine whether medications or treatment modalities contribute to the sleep complaint. If so, evaluate whether the type of medication or dosing schedule can be altered.
4. Consider the possibility of a primary sleep disorder. Formal polysomnography may be necessary.
5. Consider the sleep needs of hospitalized patients when ordering checks of vital signs and other procedures. Keep awakenings to a minimum.
6. Review principles of good sleep hygiene (see Chapter 3) with all patients.
7. Use hypnotics to treat patients with acute medical illnesses and insomnia if no contraindications exist.

■ PSYCHIATRIC DISORDERS AND SLEEP

Many psychiatric disorders are associated with prominent disturbances in sleep, most often in the form of insomnia but occasionally in the form of excessive sleepiness, nightmares, or parasomnia-type behaviors. In this section, we address the most frequently encountered sleep complaints found in the major groups of psychiatric disorders (see Tables 6–3 and 6–4). The area of sleep disorders associated with substance abuse is considered separately in Chapter 3.

The complaint of insomnia is often accompanied by some indication of psychological stress. Evaluation of large groups of patients with chronic insomnia, using the Minnesota Multiphasic Personality Inventory, has shown that as many as 75% of patients with insomnia may have some degree of depression or dysthymia, and it has been estimated that 35%–50% of chronic insomnia may be causally related to psychiatric illness. It is often not clear which comes first—the insomnia or the depression and/or anxiety. Patients often state, "You'd feel miserable and depressed too if you slept no more than I do." Similarly, it is not always clear whether anxiety precipitates insomnia or whether a period of insomnia leads

---

TABLE 6–3. **DSM-IV-TR diagnostic criteria for insomnia related to an Axis I or Axis II disorder**

A. The predominant complaint is difficulty initiating or maintaining sleep, or nonrestorative sleep, for at least 1 month that is associated with daytime fatigue or impaired daytime functioning.

B. The sleep disturbance (or daytime sequelae) causes clinically significant distress or impairment in social, occupational, or other important areas of functioning.

C. The insomnia is judged to be related to another Axis I or Axis II disorder (e.g., Major Depressive Disorder, Generalized Anxiety Disorder, Adjustment Disorder With Anxiety) but is sufficiently severe to warrant independent clinical attention.

D. The disturbance is not better accounted for by another Sleep Disorder (e.g., Narcolepsy, Breathing-Related Sleep Disorder, a Parasomnia).

E. The disturbance is not due to the direct physiological effects of a substance (e.g., a drug of abuse, a medication) or a general medical condition.

TABLE 6–4. **DSM-IV-TR diagnostic criteria for hypersomnia related to an Axis I or Axis II disorder**

A. The predominant complaint is excessive sleepiness for at least 1 month as evidenced by either prolonged sleep episodes or daytime sleep episodes that occur almost daily.

B. The excessive sleepiness causes clinically significant distress or impairment in social, occupational, or other important areas of functioning.

C. The hypersomnia is judged to be related to another Axis I or Axis II disorder (e.g., Major Depressive Disorder, Dysthymic Disorder) but is sufficiently severe to warrant independent clinical attention.

D. The disturbance is not better accounted for by another Sleep Disorder (e.g., Narcolepsy, Breathing-Related Sleep Disorder, a Parasomnia) or by an inadequate amount of sleep.

E. The disturbance is not due to the direct physiological effects of a substance (e.g., a drug of abuse, a medication) or a general medical condition.

---

to anxiety about going to bed, only to lie awake and be unable to sleep. Such concerns underscore the importance of a thorough psychiatric evaluation as a part of a sleep history.

Psychiatric Assessment

Many of the important psychological variables can be elicited subtly during the interview by asking open-ended questions in areas such as current stressful events in the patient's life or events that may have occurred around the time of initial insomnia. The clinician should also evaluate premorbid psychological and physical functioning. It is important to ask questions about childhood sleeping patterns. Doing so can also elicit information about possible early developmental conflicts. Many patients fear being labeled a "psychiatric patient." They may have biases that lead them to believe that if their sleep complaint is caused by something that is "all in your head," it is not truly a valid complaint. These patients may consequently steer away from talking about their depression or anxiety-related symptoms.

The clinician should begin the interview by creating avenues for patients to express their concerns openly and then should proceed to ask difficult questions directly: Have suicidal ideas crossed your mind while lying awake? Have hopelessness and despondency set in around the fears of being unable to control insomnia? Have you had episodes of anxiety with physical symptoms such as tachycardia or hyperventilation? For many patients, the direct questions about symptoms of depression or panic disorder may relieve their fear of bringing up symptoms that they feel the physician may not want to hear or are "too crazy to talk about."

The clinician usually should refrain from drawing diagnostic conclusions on the basis of information obtained during the first visit. We find that many times, patients are indeed correct in that their mood disorder symptoms or anxiety is secondary to their insomnia and that these symptoms may resolve with treatment of the sleep complaint. If the clinician finds that psychiatric symptoms persist after appropriate behavioral and pharmacological intervention, he or she may speculate that the psychiatric symptoms are likely to be primary and need their own specific treatment plan.

Psychiatric Disorders Associated Primarily With Insomnia

The following psychiatric disorders (listed in Table 6–5) are those most frequently associated with insomnia.

Schizophrenia

Deterioration of sleep, including a marked increase in frequency of nightmares, is common in schizophrenic patients before a psychotic break. Sleep EEGs have shown a tendency toward sleep fragmentation and a decrease in slow-wave sleep in most patients with schizophrenia. Acute schizophrenia has also been associated with shortened REM sleep latency. In general, however, no diagnostically specific sleep EEG abnormalities are found in schizophrenia.

TABLE 6–5. **Psychiatric disorders frequently associated with sleep complaints**

Psychiatric disorders associated with insomnia

Schizophrenia
Major depression
Bipolar disorder
Dysthymic disorder
Cyclothymic disorder
Personality disorders
Anxiety disorders
    Panic disorder
    Generalized anxiety disorder
    Obsessive-compulsive disorder
Other disorders
    Somatoform disorders
    Posttraumatic stress disorder

Psychiatric disorders associated with excessive daytime sleepiness

Seasonal affective disorders
Atypical depression

The preferred treatment of schizophrenia-related insomnia is administration of a neuroleptic that will stabilize the psychotic symptoms and offer enough sedation to provide adequate sleep. Newer-generation or atypical antipsychotics are antagonists of the serotonin-2 receptor (Jibson and Tandon 1998). This postsynaptic receptor is involved in control of anxiety, depression, psychosis, sleep, and migraines. These antipsychotics appear to be more effective in controlling psychosis and insomnia, with fewer side effects than traditional dopamine antagonists, although at times they can be too sedating. When choosing an antipsychotic, the clinician should consider the dual needs of reducing psychosis and providing appropriate sedation. It is preferable to avoid adding benzodiazepines to the neuroleptic for long-term use. Table 6–6 includes examples of antipsychotic drugs.

TABLE 6–6. **Sedative antipsychotics**

Agent	Dose range (mg)
Dopamine antagonists	
Perphenazine	4–64
Loxapine	10–250
Thioridazine	25–800
Chlorpromazine	25–800
Serotonin antagonists	
Clozapine	25–600
Risperidone	0.5–20
Olanzapine	5–20
Quetiapine	25–600
Ziprasidone	40–160

It is important to note sleep problems that may develop later in the lives of patients with schizophrenia. The clinician should determine whether this sleep deterioration is a side effect of medication or evidence of poor control of the psychosis, onset of depression, or emergence of a specific sleep syndrome such as sleep apnea. Patients with chronic schizophrenia who undergo long-term drug therapy may gain an excessive amount of weight as a result of appetite stimulation and may develop obstructive sleep apnea secondary to this weight gain. In these patients, interventions such as weight loss, nasal CPAP therapy, or even surgery may be required.

Major Depression

Nearly 20% of Americans will have an episode of major depression during their adult lives, and 90%–95% of these people will have disordered sleep during this bout of depression (Buysse et al. 1994). Insomnia is the most frequent sleep complaint and appears as sleep-onset insomnia, frequent awakenings, nonrestorative sleep, or early-morning awakenings with difficulty returning to sleep.

   The insomnia of major depression has a very high likelihood of response to antidepressants, so it is important to keep the diagnostic criteria in mind. A useful mnemonic for the symptoms of depression is D SIG ECAPS, which is a reminder that the prescription for *D*epression would be written *SIG: E*(nergy) *CAPS*(ules) (see Table 6–7).

   The presence of five of these nine symptoms for 2 weeks or more, including the presence of either depressed mood or loss of interest, fulfills the criteria for the diagnosis of major depression.

TABLE 6–7. **Mnemonic for diagnosis of depression: D SIG ECAPS**

Depressed mood

Sleeplessness

Interests—decreased

Guilt—increased

Energy—decreased

Concentration—decreased

Appetite—diminished

Psychomotor agitation or retardation

Suicidal ideation

Nocturnal polysomnographic studies in depressed patients show a tendency toward decreased sleep continuity, decreased delta sleep, and decreased nocturnal REM sleep latency (time between sleep onset and onset of the first REM sleep period). Phasic activity (e.g., REM density), the duration of the first REM sleep period, and total REM sleep may increase. Thus, REM sleep occurs earlier and is more intense in patients with major depression than in nondepressed subjects. It is similar to nondepressed individuals' REM sleep in the early-morning hours. These findings have suggested that the REM sleep rhythm may be phase-advanced in major depression. It has also been postulated that depression is associated with a relative increase in central cholinergic activity compared with monoaminergic activity; cholinergic systems have been shown to reduce slow-wave sleep and increase REM sleep.

The sleep EEG has been a helpful tool in predicting response to medication. Patients with major depression or subaffective disorders who have shortened REM sleep latencies, which increase in length with the administration of tricyclic antidepressants, are more likely to respond positively to tricyclic antidepressants than are patients with normal REM sleep latencies. Short REM sleep latency and deficits in slow-wave sleep appear to be familial. Short REM sleep latency is associated with an increased risk of major depression beyond the expected familial risk associated with a depressed proband (Giles et al. 1998). Still, many other psychiatric illnesses show similar sleep disturbances, and patients with severe depression may show no sleep EEG abnormalities. This, plus expense, has greatly limited the usefulness of sleep EEGs in diagnosis and treatment of mood disorders.

Major depression with insomnia should be treated with pharmacotherapy and/or psychotherapy to alleviate the depressive symptoms. As the depression improves, sleep tends to improve as well, and the latter improvement serves as a marker of progress.

Many antidepressants are quite effective for depression. Their antidepressant effects appear to be independent of their effects on sleep. The effects of antidepressant agents on polysomnographically determined sleep patterns, as well as the sedative properties of these agents, are tabulated in Table 6–8. Serotonin reuptake inhibitors and venlafaxine are the most commonly prescribed first-line agents for treatment of depression. At times, these drugs can trigger multiple microarousals and aggravate sleep quality and efficiency. Adjunctive use of hypnotic agents or sedating antidepressants such as trazodone or mirtazapine can improve sleep quality and at times enhance antidepressant response. Serotonin-2 antagonist drugs such as nefazodone or mirtazapine may at times be appropriate first-line agents in serious insomnia, given their tendency to improve sleep quality (Gursky and Krahn 2000; Oberndorfer et al. 2000; Rush et al. 1998; Thase 1999).

Tricyclic antidepressants promote improved sleep, but their toxicity in overdose and anticholinergic side effects have relegated these to a secondary role. Monoamine oxidase inhibitors (MAOIs) may be good choices for patients with treatment-resistant depression or with atypical bipolar depressions unresponsive to serotonin reuptake inhibitors.

If depression is reduced and sleep improves, medication should be continued at the same doses for 6 months, and then use of the medication should be reevaluated. Some investigators have proposed that one episode of depression after age 50, two episodes after age 40, or three or more episodes at any age are good reason to continue maintenance antidepressant therapy indefinitely.

If depression is reduced but sleep remains impaired, the clinician would consider the following differential diagnosis: 1) the antidepressant's stimulating or sleep-disruptive properties prevent adequate sleep (e.g., akathisia, nocturnal arousals, periodic leg movements), 2) only a partial response has been obtained, or 3) the patient has switched into hypomania or mania.

If sleep improves but depression is persistent, the clinician can increase the antidepressant dose, add an augmenting agent, or switch to an alternative antidepressant.

Also, it is often necessary to help the patient cope with negatively conditioned or psychophysiological aspects of his or her sleep disturbance by promoting sleep hygiene or sleep-restriction programs. Concurrent psychotherapy for the depressed patient is

TABLE 6–8.   Overview of effects of antidepressants on sleep

Drug	Sleep EEG effects			
	Continuity	SWS	REM sleep	Sedation
Tricyclic antidepressants				
Amitriptyline	↑↑↑	↑	↓↓↓	++++
Doxepin	↑↑↑	↑↑	↓↓	++++
Imipramine	↔↑	↑	↓↓	++
Nortriptyline	↑	↑	↓↓	++
Desipramine	↔	↑	↓↓	+
Clomipramine	↑↔	↑	↓↓↓↓	±
MAOIs				
Phenelzine	↓	↔	↓↓↓↓	↔
Tranylcypromine	↓↓	↔	↓↓↓↓	↔
SSRIs				
Fluoxetine	↓	↔↓	↔↓	±
Paroxetine[a]	↓	↔↓	↓↓	±
Sertraline	↔	↔	↓↓	↔
Citalopram	↓	↔	↓	ND
Fluvoxamine	↓	↔	↓	ND
Other antidepressants				
Bupropion	↓↔	↔	↑	↔
Venlafaxine	↓	↓	↓↓↓	++
Trazodone	↑↑↑	↔↑	↓	++++
Mirtazapine	↑↑↑	↑↑	↔	+++
Nefazodone	↑	↔	↑	+

Note.   ↑=increased; ↓=decreased; ↔=no change; +=slight effect; ++=small effect; +++=moderate effect; ++++=great effect; ±=no significant effect.
EEG=electroencephalogram; MAOI=monoamine oxidase inhibitor; ND=no data available; REM=rapid eye movement; SSRI=selective serotonin reuptake inhibitor; SWS=slow-wave sleep.
[a]When taken at bedtime, paroxetine potentially decreases sleep continuity less than other SSRIs.
Source.   Adapted from Winokur A, Reynolds C: "Overview of Effects of Antidepressant Therapies on Sleep." *Primary Psychiatry* 1:22–27, 1994. Used with permission.

often helpful as well. It should combine supportive and cognitive elements to help the patient work through loss or bereavement issues, identify and explain maladaptive patterns, boost self-esteem, appropriately express anger, and decrease the tendency toward self-criticism.

Patients whose depression is resistant to treatment may also benefit from the sedative properties of valproate, mood stabilizers such as carbamazepine, or atypical antipsychotics such as quetiapine or olanzapine.

Dysthymic Disorder

Dysthymic disorder is diagnosed by noting the presence of at least 2 years of depressed mood accompanied by symptoms such as abnormal sleep, abnormal appetite, decreased energy, decreased self-esteem, hopelessness, and poor concentration. Approximately half of patients with dysthymic disorder complain of insomnia. Research indicates that dysthymic patients respond to psychotherapy and antidepressant medications in a way similar to that in which patients with major depression respond.

Bipolar Disorders

In the acute manic phase, patients with bipolar disorder have sharply reduced sleep times, but they may have a great deal of energy despite the minimal amount of sleep. Sleep studies suggest that sleep during the manic phase may involve changes in REM and slow-wave sleep similar to those seen in depression. During the depressed phases, these same patients may exhibit hypersomnia but still complain of fatigue and lethargy. Appropriate regulation of sleep in the bipolar patient is important because sleep deprivation can trigger manic episodes and deter mood stabilization (Wehr et al. 1987). During the acute phase, the use of benzodiazepines and/or mood stabilizers with sedative properties is usually the most effective treatment for the sleep problem until the patient can be stabilized with an antimanic drug such as lithium, divalproex, or carbamazepine. Atypical neuroleptics such as olanzapine and quetiapine are now commonly used in both acute and maintenance treatment of bipolar disorders. They have relatively benign side effects and provide mood stabilization, sedation, and the opportunity for rapid increases without fear of severe toxicity. Typical neuroleptics can provide sedation as well but should be reserved for patients with psychotic symptoms.

Bipolar disorder is now diagnosed more frequently since the evidence of its frequent presentation with hypomania alternating with major depression (bipolar II disorder), simultaneous depression and mania/hypomania (mixed bipolar disorder), irritability without euphoria (dysphoric mania), and hypomania alternating with dysthymia (cyclothymic disorder). These more subtle presentations led to the designation of bipolar disorder as a *spectrum disorder*. Many of these more subtle bipolar disorders can be detected in patients with treatment-resistant depression or marginal or adverse responses to antidepressants.

To diagnose any sleep problem or mood disorder, the clinician should quickly assess the patient for diagnostic criteria for bipolar disorder. We find it beneficial to use the mnemonic IE RATE DIS, which emphasizes that bipolar disorder is an IE (i.e.—that is) RATE DIS(order), or a disorder with variable rates of activity, thinking, talking, and responding (see Table 6–9). The diagnosis of mania is determined by the presence of euphoria or irritability for a period of at least 7 days. If euphoria is present, three of the secondary (RATE DIS) criteria also must be fulfilled. If only irritability is present, four of the secondary criteria must be met.

The clinician must keep a number of important facts in mind when evaluating poor responses to antidepressants and when considering the diagnosis of bipolar spectrum disorders:

- Bipolar disorder can develop later in life and may initially present as recurrent unipolar depression in the patient's 20s and 30s.
- Two of three bipolar patients abuse substances, and manic or hypomanic states may be obscured by substance abuse.
- Hypomanic states can often be quite pleasurable and productive and are not seen as pathological for many years.

TABLE 6–9. **Mnemonic for diagnosis of bipolar disorder: IE RATE DIS**

Irritability

Euphoria, elation, expansive mood (One of these must be present for 4 days for a diagnosis of hypomania or 7 days for a diagnosis of mania.)

Risky or dangerous behavior

Activity level—increased

Talkativeness—increased

Esteem—elevated (grandiosity)

Distractibility

Idea flight or racing thoughts

Sleep disturbance, generally insomnia or a decreased need for sleep

- If untreated, bipolar disorder tends to result in an increase in frequency and severity of episodes over time.
- Antidepressant medications may intensify mania and destabilize mood in bipolar patients.

Investigators have noted that antidepressants that induce stimulation may worsen the life course of bipolar disorder and possibly induce rapidly alternating mood cycles or mixed bipolar states. See Table 6–10 for doses and sedative properties of currently used anticycling agents.

TABLE 6–10. **Sedative properties of mood stabilizers**

Drug	Dose range (mg)	Sedation
Lithium carbonate	300–2,400	Weak
Divalproex	125–5,000	Moderate
Carbamazepine	100–2,000	Strong
Verapamil	160–480	Weak
Gabapentin	300–4,800	Moderate to strong
Oxcarbazepine	150–2,400	Strong
Tiagabine	4–32	Moderate
Lamotrigine	25–600	Moderate
Topiramate	25–400	Moderate

When prescribing medication to help patients with bipolar disorder sleep, the clinician should 1) never use antidepressants merely for their sedative properties (if antidepressants are necessary for persistent depression after a manic patient is stabilized, he or she should use nonstimulating selective serotonin reuptake inhibitors, bupropion, or MAOIs, but not tricyclics); 2) use benzodiazepines such as clonazepam and lorazepam for acute stabilization and occasionally for maintenance treatment for persistent insomnia or anxiety but should avoid using them over the long run in patients with histories of substance abuse; 3) use an additional mood stabilizer for both its sedative properties and adjunctive mood stabilization; and 4) use one of the more sedating drugs such as carbamazepine or gabapentin or a primary augmenting agent if insomnia is a particularly problematic aspect of the bipolar disorder (Schatzberg and Nemeroff 2001).

Personality Disorders

REM sleep latency has often been found to be decreased in patients with borderline personality disorder studied with polysomnography. Patients with shortened REM sleep latencies were more likely to respond to tricyclic antidepressants, with benefits in both mood and sleep, than were patients with normal REM sleep latencies. Thus, we now carefully screen all patients with personality disorders for concurrent mood disorders. Appropriate treatment of mood instability and sleep problems can often reduce or eliminate many symptoms thought to be part of a character disorder. These patients may often benefit from administration of mood stabilizers, antidepressants, or atypical neuroleptics. Newer atypical neuroleptics are likely to see increasing use in this population.

Anxiety Disorders

Anxiety disorders are one of the most common health problems in the United States, with a lifetime prevalence of about 8%.

Panic disorder is the most severe anxiety disorder. It is diagnosed by noting the presence of four or more panic attacks in a

4-week period. The attacks must begin spontaneously or without the presence of a situation that typically produces anxiety. To qualify as a panic attack, an episode must contain four or more symptoms from a list that includes tachycardia, shortness of breath, chest pain or discomfort, sweating, choking, dizziness or faintness, nausea, depersonalization, paresthesias, tremulousness, fear of dying, hot flushes or chills, and fear of going crazy. Panic disorder can be accompanied by agoraphobia (i.e., avoidance of unprotected situations, especially those that may be associated with previous panic attacks). Milder forms of panic can occur with fewer than four symptoms (panic disorder symptom attacks), which may still be quite incapacitating.

Sleep disturbances, predominantly insomnia, are extremely common in patients with panic disorder. Complaints include initial, middle, and late insomnia as well as nocturnal or sleep panic attacks. Initial insomnia can be quite severe in patients with evening panic and symptom attacks, and sleep panic attacks tend to cause paralyzed awakenings at night. Many patients with panic disorder experience occasional sleep panic attacks, but only about 30%–45% of patients with panic disorder have repeated sleep panic attacks (Benca 1996). Those with frequent sleep panic attacks have a severe form of panic disorder that is correlated with a greater frequency of depression and sleep disruption as well as a greater sensitivity to attacks that are triggered by relaxation or sleep deprivation. Some patients with sleep panic attacks can develop a conditioned fear or even an avoidance of sleep, which may cause further sleep deprivation and thus aggravate the condition.

Polysomnographic studies indicate that patients with panic disorders have surprisingly normal sleep patterns. They have a moderate tendency toward increased sleep latency, reduced sleep efficiency, and increased body movements. Sleep panic attacks appear to occur frequently during the transition from Stage II to Stage III sleep. Some patients have panic attacks exclusively during sleep. Nocturnal polysomnography is generally recommended to rule out sleep apnea, parasomnia, or other primary sleep disorders.

Treatment generally consists of both pharmacological and behavioral interventions.

Research suggests that panic disorder responds to a number of pharmacological agents, including selective serotonin reuptake inhibitors, tricyclic antidepressants, benzodiazepines, and MAOIs. Because patients with panic disorder are quite sensitive to stimulation, they initially may have increased anxiety or insomnia in response to antidepressant medications. This response should alert the clinician to increase the dose quite slowly and can be a reason to use a benzodiazepine, to reduce anxiety and aid sleep, in the early phase of treatment. Approximately 25%–35% of patients with panic disorder do not respond to antidepressants alone and may require ongoing use of benzodiazepines. Some patients have panic attacks or symptom attacks only in the evening or at night. They often have a primary complaint of insomnia and appear to respond quite well to a once-a-day dose of an intermediate-half-life benzodiazepine.

Generalized anxiety disorder is characterized by chronic worry with somatic symptoms of anxiety, and the symptoms do not meet criteria for another DSM-IV-TR Axis I disorder. Many patients with generalized anxiety disorder complain of insomnia. Polysomnographic studies support the presence of increased sleep latencies, increased wake time, and reduced delta slow-wave sleep in these patients.

Generalized anxiety disorder is often responsive to benzodiazepines, buspirone, and antidepressants. Adjunctive psychotherapy with a cognitive focus can be beneficial. Often, alleviation of the sleep disturbance can greatly improve the condition; therefore, a low-dose intermediate-acting benzodiazepine at bedtime may be temporarily indicated early in treatment.

Obsessive-compulsive disorder (OCD) has a lifetime prevalence in the population of about 2.5%. It is diagnosed by noting obsessions or compulsions that cause a significant disruption in a person's daily routine. *Obsessions* are defined in DSM-IV-TR as recurrent and persistent ideas, thoughts, impulses, or images that are experienced, at least initially, as senseless and intrusive (e.g., fear that one has hit someone with one's car). *Compulsions* are repetitive, purposeful, and intentional behaviors linked to an obsession that are performed in a stereotypical way. Examples of compulsions are driving around the block to see whether someone was hit by one's car, washing one's hands repeatedly, or performing elaborate behavioral rituals before going to bed.

In patients with OCD, polysomnographic studies indicate a tendency toward decreased sleep efficiency, decreased total sleep time, decreased deep sleep, shortened REM sleep latency, and increased REM density, a pattern quite similar to that of major depression. Subjectively, patients with OCD often complain of disrupted sleep and sleep delay related to compulsive behaviors.

Treatment is generally a combination of pharmacotherapy with serotonin-potentiating agents and behavior therapy. The most frequently used medications are clomipramine, fluoxetine, fluvoxamine, and other serotonin reuptake inhibitors. These drugs are generally started at low doses and gradually increased to doses significantly above those used for depression (e.g., fluoxetine 60–80 mg/day). Because fluoxetine or fluvoxamine can be stimulating and induce insomnia, the concurrent use of trazodone (a mild serotonin potentiator that is ineffective for OCD on its own) at bedtime is often prescribed. Concurrent behavior therapy techniques include thought stopping, exposure treatment, systematic desensitization, cognitive therapy, and response prevention.

Somatoform Disorder

The patient who somatizes appears to convert an emotional problem into a physical complaint. Insomnia as a somatized complaint is probably second in frequency only to headaches. The typical patient with somatoform disorder will actually have a broad array of physical complaints, which become quite fixed over time and for which no underlying medical illness, positive laboratory test results, or adequate treatment can be found. These patients are very poor at articulating their emotions and may exhibit alexithymia (i.e., an inability to express emotions).

Many of these patients have grown up in an environment of physical or emotional abuse or neglect, and symptoms may be the patients' perceived link to a source of caring or concern. These patients may become angry if the physician tries to reassure them that they are "going to be all right." Attempts to minimize the seriousness of their illness may only increase the tenacity with which these patients cling to the symptoms. It is very important in the case of patients with somatoform disorder not to prescribe sleeping medications without having a very clear understanding about when, and for how long, the medications will be prescribed. If the physician believes that the sleeping medication is not likely to solve the problem, it is best not to administer medication. The clinician should express to the patient that he or she recognizes the patient's frustration with the illness and that he or she respects the treatments the patient has received and will not abruptly change any current medication regimens. Regular follow-up appointments should be scheduled.

Posttraumatic Stress Disorder

Posttraumatic stress disorder (PTSD) is a syndrome of anxiety and chronic hyperarousal related to preoccupation with and reexperiencing of severely traumatic or life-threatening events such as war experiences, serious accidents, and physical or sexual assaults. PTSD is often characterized by repetitive traumatic memories of the original event, preoccupation with the original trauma, and frequent reexposure to the traumatic event through flashbacks, nightmares, and night terrors (Lavie 2001). Chronic insomnia secondary to the hyperarousal is very common. Patients with PTSD may become socially isolated and, at times, may resort to the use of drugs or alcohol to suppress the traumatic memories and tormented wakefulness.

Nocturnal PSG of a patient with PTSD is characterized by shortened sleep time, frequent awakenings, and frequent night terror–type arousals from slow-wave sleep. Most of these night terror–type events occur during the first third of the night, and they are often accompanied by verbalization, emotion, and more dreamlike content than is usually seen in night terrors. Nightmares are associated with REM sleep and generally occur later in the night.

Most patients with PTSD can benefit from some form of psychotherapy, either individual or group, especially early in the course of the syndrome. Talking about their traumatic experiences seems to be quite helpful and may, over time, diminish the continued anxiety and hyperarousal. Early in treatment, in very severe cases, medication is usually necessary to suppress night terror activity, suppress nightmares during REM sleep, and help provide relief for the chronic insomnia. Tricyclic antidepressants, at antidepressant doses, have historically been the most common mode of treatment. Other medications that have frequently been useful in treating PTSD include MAOIs, carbamazepine, lithium, cyproheptadine, propranolol, divalproex, fluoxetine, sertraline, nefazodone, and other antidepressants. The overdose potential of tricyclics has led to more common use of serotonin reuptake inhibitors. Hyperarousal states may benefit from the use of adrenergic blockers (e.g., clonidine or propranolol), anticonvulsants (e.g., divalproex or carbamazepine), or atypical neuroleptics (e.g., quetiapine or olanzapine). Typical neuroleptics are only appropriate if the patient has prominent hallucinations or paranoia. Cyproheptadine (16–24 mg) has been shown to block combat nightmares. Benzodiazepines may be helpful, but tolerance may develop because of the disorder's chronicity. Another reason to be cautious when using benzodiazepines is the common concurrence of substance use disorders and PTSD.

Psychiatric Disorders Associated With Excessive Daytime Sleepiness

Seasonal Affective Disorders

Seasonal affective disorders (SADs) are disorders of mood, presenting as depression, hypomania, or mania, that are very closely linked to certain seasons. SADs may be related to a circadian rhythm disturbance precipitated by changes in the length of the day. A typical example is a woman in her 30s who begins to show evidence of depression and excessive sleepiness in October and November (in the Northern Hemisphere). The depression might last throughout the winter and only begin to improve as the days become longer in the spring. Most of the depressive symptoms tend to be atypical, with increased sleep time, decreased energy, increased appetite and carbohydrate craving, increased weight, decreased activity, and increased daytime drowsiness. Some patients report the opposite symptoms in the spring and summer, with the development of hypomanic symptoms, including irritability, decreased sleep, and hyperactivity.

SAD is diagnosed in patients who have had at least one major depressive episode and who have had at least two occurrences of fall/winter depression, with nondepressed periods during the spring and summer. In addition to this typical SAD, a reverse SAD that consists of a hypomanic period during the winter and a period of depression during the spring and summer apparently exists. Patients with spring/summer depression, however, appear to report decreased sleep and decreased appetite. No clear polysomnographic findings seem to identify SAD.

Patients with SADs have been found to respond to bright light exposure (via a light box, at least 30 minutes at 10,000 lux) immediately on awakening in the morning. Commercial light units are available to provide this high-intensity light. The unit is normally placed about 1–2 feet in front of the patient so that the light falls on the retina. The patient does not look directly at the light but is instructed to glance at the light once per minute. Light treatment should begin 3 hours after midpoint of habitual sleep. Response should occur within a few days and should be complete within 2 weeks (Neson and Oren 2001; Terman et al. 2001). If the patient does not respond to treatment, the clinician should consider increasing light exposure or shifting light exposure to evening hours. A patient with SAD who has early-morning awakening should begin his or her trial of light exposure in the evening. Psychotropic drugs such as antidepressants, MAOIs, lithium, divalproex, and carbamazepine may be useful treatment adjuncts. In one study, winter depression was successfully treated with ingestion of melatonin in the afternoon (Lewy et al. 1998). The underlying mood disorder may be either unipolar or bipolar and should be carefully evaluated independent of the seasonal variation.

Atypical Depression

Atypical depression differs from the usual presentation of major depression in that patients tend to have excessive sleepiness, lethargy (often appearing as "leaden paralysis"), increased appetite, carbohydrate craving, rejection sensitivity, and an inability to initiate enjoyable activities, despite an ability to enjoy pleasurable activities initiated by others (mood reactivity). Symptoms in common with major depression include poor concentration, decreased energy, low self-esteem, and suicidal ideation.

Atypical depression is often responsive to MAOIs such as phenelzine. MAOIs tend to be somewhat activating and may reduce sleep time, which can be beneficial for patients with excessive sleep as a presenting complaint. Activating serotonin reuptake inhibitors, such as fluoxetine, paroxetine, and venlafaxine, are often effective as well.

The clinician should remember that major depression can also present with hypersomnolence and that defense mechanisms found in many psychiatric disorders can include hypersomnolence and drowsiness as a form of psychological withdrawal. Also, atypical depressions are commonly seen in the depressed phase of a bipolar disorder. Patients with atypical depression should always be assessed carefully for personal and family histories of mania, hypomania, or cyclical mood disturbances. Often these patients require mood stabilizers plus antidepressants.

■ REFERENCES

American Psychiatric Association: Diagnostic and Statistical Manual of Mental Disorders, 4th Edition, Text Revision. Washington, DC, American Psychiatric Association, 2000

Benca R: Sleep in psychotic disorders. Neurol Clin 14:739–764, 1996

Buysse DJ, Reynolds CF 3rd, Kupfer DJ, et al: Clinical diagnoses in 216 insomnia patients using the International Classification of Sleep Disorders (ICSD), DSM-IV and ICD-10 categories: a report from the APA/NIMH DSM-IV Field Trial. Sleep 17:630–637, 1994

Fein AM, Niederman MS, Imbriano L, et al: Reversal of sleep apnea in uremia by dialysis. Arch Intern Med 147:1355–1356, 1987

Giles EG, Kupfer DJ, Rush AJ, et al: Controlled comparison of electrophysiological sleep in families of probands with unipolar depression. Am J Psychiatry 155:192–199, 1998

Gursky JT, Krahn LE: The effects of antidepressants on sleep: a review. Harv Rev Psychiatry 8:298–306, 2000

Harding SM: Sleep in fibromyalgia patients: subjective and objective findings. Am J Med Sci 315:367–376, 1998

Javaheri S, Parker TJ, Wexler L, et al: Occult sleep-disordered breathing in stable congestive heart failure. Ann Intern Med 122:487–492, 1995

Jibson MD, Tandon R: New atypical antipsychotic medications. J Psychiatr Res 32:215–228, 1998

Krupp LB, Jandorf L, Coyle PK, et al: Sleep disturbance in chronic fatigue syndrome. J Psychosom Res 37:325–331, 1993

Langevin B, Fouque D, Leger P, et al: Sleep apnea syndrome and end-stage renal disease: cure after renal transplantation. Chest 103:1330–1335, 1993

Lavie P: Sleep disturbances in the wake of traumatic events. N Engl J Med 345:1825–1832, 2001

Lewy AJ, Bauer VK, Cutler NL, et al: Melatonin treatment of winter depression: a pilot study. Psychiatry Res 77:57–61, 1998

Mendelson W, Wadhwa NK, Greenberg HE, et al: Effects of hemodialysis on sleep apnea syndrome in end-stage renal disease. Clin Nephrol 33:247–251, 1990

Montagna P, Cortelli P, Gambetti P, et al: Fatal familial insomnia: sleep, neuroendocrine and vegetative alterations. Adv Neuroimmunol 5:13–21, 1995

Munschauer FE, Loh L, Bannister R, et al: Abnormal respiration and sudden death during sleep in multiple system atrophy with autonomic failure. Neurology 40:677–679, 1990

Naughton MT, Bernard DC, Rutherford R, et al: Effect of continuous positive airway pressure on central sleep apnea and nocturnal pCO_2 in heart failure. Am J Respir Crit Care Med 150:1598–1604, 1994

Neson P, Oren D: Is seasonal affective disorder a disorder of circadian rhythms? CNS Spectrums 6:487–501, 2001

Norman SE, Chediak AD, Freeman C, et al: Sleep disturbances in men with asymptomatic human immunodeficiency (HIV) infection. Sleep 15:150–155, 1992

Oberndorfer S, Saletu-Zyhlarz G, Saletu B: Effects of selective serotonin reuptake inhibitors on objective and subjective sleep quality. Neuropsychobiology 42:69–81, 2000

Rush AJ, Armitage K, Gillin JC, et al: Comparative effects of nefazodone and fluoxetine on sleep in outpatients with major depressive disorder. Biol Psychiatry 44:3–14, 1998

Schatzberg AF, Nemeroff CB (eds): Essentials of Clinical Psychopharmacology. Washington, DC, American Psychiatric Publishing, 2001

Sin DD, Logan AG, Fitzgerald FS, et al: Effects of continuous positive airway pressure on cardiovascular outcomes in heart failure patients with and without Cheyne-Stokes respiration. Circulation 102:61–66, 2000

Terman JS, Terman M, Lo ES, et al: Circadian time of morning light administration and therapeutic response in winter depression. Arch Gen Psychiatry 58:69–75, 2001

Thase ME: Antidepressant treatment of the depressed patient with insomnia. J Clin Psychiatry 60(suppl 17):28–31, 1999

VanDyck P, Chadband R, Chaudhary B, et al: Sleep apnea, sleep disorders, and hypothyroidism. Am J Med Sci 298:119–122, 1989

Wehr TA, Sack DA, Rosenthal NE: Sleep reduction as a final common pathway in the genesis of mania. Am J Psychiatry 144:201–204, 1987

MEDICATIONS WITH SEDATIVE-HYPNOTIC PROPERTIES

Sedative-hypnotic drugs are among the most widely prescribed medications today. Sedative drugs moderate excitement and induce calmness, and hypnotic drugs promote drowsiness and facilitate the onset of sleep. Benzodiazepines and the benzodiazepine receptor agonists zaleplon and zolpidem are currently the most commonly used sedative-hypnotics. In addition, antidepressants, mood stabilizers, antipsychotics, and a number of over-the-counter agents are valuable for their sedative-hypnotic properties in specific situations. Historically, agents such as chloral hydrate, paraldehyde, barbiturates, glutethimide, methyprylon, and meprobamate were used as hypnotics. Although the rare continuing clinical utility of these agents is still covered in comprehensive pharmacology textbooks, we believe that these agents have no current clinical use in the long-term management of chronic insomnia. Improved efficacy and side-effect profiles have propelled benzodiazepine-1 receptor agonists to the forefront in current hypnotic prescribing. Mendelson and Jain (1995) suggest that the ideal hypnotic would have the profiles listed in Table 7–1. The perfect hypnotic, according to these criteria, has not been developed, but some of the newer agents, such as zolpidem and zaleplon, appear to be approaching this ideal.

■ HYPNOTICS FOR TRANSIENT INSOMNIA

Properly used, recently developed hypnotic agents can provide marked relief of insomnia symptoms in most patients in many

TABLE 7–1. **Therapeutic and pharmacological profiles of an "ideal" hypnotic**

Therapeutic profile
Rapid sleep induction
No residual effects
No effect on memory

Pharmacokinetic profile
Rapid absorption
Specific receptor binding
Optimal half-life
No active metabolites

Pharmacodynamic profile
No tolerance
No physical dependence
No respiratory or central nervous system depression

diverse settings, and there is evidence of good efficacy, good margin of safety with minimal risk, and very little abuse potential.

The proper use of hypnotics to enhance sleep can greatly improve daytime functioning by decreasing fatigue, improving concentration and memory, and promoting an enhanced sense of well-being. Untreated insomnia can greatly increase the likelihood of traffic and work-related accidents, significantly impair performance on many levels, and impair overall functioning and well-being. The extent to which these drugs are underused is related primarily to fears of overprescribing and addiction.

Guidelines that were established by a 1984 National Institute of Mental Health consensus study on insomnia encouraged proper use of sedative-hypnotics. Benzodiazepines were then recommended as the drugs of choice for transient insomnia, and prescribing the lowest effective dose for the shortest possible time was encouraged. Most important, the guidelines emphasized careful assessment and treatment of underlying causes of insomnia (discussed in Chapters 3 and 6). The comprehensive and accurate differential diagnosis of an insomnia complaint remains equally important today as in 1984, although current hypnotic agents are safer and more effective than those used in the past. Table 7–2 lists numerous sedative-hypnotic drugs, along with several of their pharmacological properties.

The most pertinent characteristics of a hypnotic are 1) the rate of absorption, 2) the rapidity of distribution in the body and central nervous system (CNS), 3) the affinity for specific CNS receptors, 4) the length of the elimination half-life, and 5) the rate of metabolic transformation. When only one or two doses are being prescribed, the first three characteristics are the most important, because they determine rate of onset duration and intensity of effect. With longer-term use, the last two characteristics are most important, because they determine potential for buildup of blood level and potential toxicity. Drugs such as diazepam have long half-lives but are so rapidly distributed in the body that the duration of action is relatively short. In elderly patients and patients with liver disease, prolongation of elimination and secondary accumulation can occur. Increased levels of benzodiazepines in elderly patients can increase the risk of falls and hip fractures, which is a seriously incapacitating problem. Drugs such as temazepam, lorazepam, and oxazepam do not require liver hydroxylation, so the metabolism rate is not prolonged in patients with decreased liver function.

Benzodiazepines

Benzodiazepines act on the inhibitory neurotransmitter receptors that are directly activated by the amino acid γ-aminobutyric acid (GABA). The major GABA receptor, $GABA_A$, is a membrane chloride channel involved in mediating most of the rapid inhibitory neurotransmission in the CNS. Typically, benzodiazepines increase the amount of chloride current at the $GABA_A$ receptor in the presence of GABA. Their effects can be blocked by the antagonist flumazenil, which is used for reversing benzodiazepine effects.

The $GABA_A$ receptor has multiple forms based on various combinations of its several subunits. Different benzodiazepines may selectively activate specific $GABA_A$ forms, which accounts for slight differences in pharmacological activity.

TABLE 7–2. Commonly used drugs with sedative-hypnotic properties, listed by half-life

Drug	Type	Half-life (hours)	Absorption	Typical dose (mg)	Active metabolite
Zolpidem (Ambien)	Imidazopyridine	1.5–4	Fast	2.5–10	No
Triazolam (Halcion)	Benzodiazepine	2–5	Fast	0.125–0.25	No
Zopliconeª	Cyclopyrrolone	5–6	Fast	3.75–7.5	Yes
Zaleplon (Sonata)	Pyrazolopyrimidine	1–1.5	Fast	5–20	No
Temazepam (Restoril)	Benzodiazepine	8–12	Moderate	7.5–30	No
Estazolam (ProSom)	Benzodiazepine	12–20	Moderate	1–2	Minimal
Oxazepam (Serax)	Benzodiazepine	5–15	Moderate	10–30	No
Alprazolam (Xanax)	Benzodiazepine	12–20	Fast	0.25–1.0	Yes
Lorazepam (Ativan)	Benzodiazepine	10–22	Moderate	0.5–2	No
Clonazepam (Klonopin)	Benzodiazepine	22–38	Slow	0.5–2	No
Diazepam (Valium)	Benzodiazepine	20–50	Fast	2.5–10	Yes
Clorazepate (Tranxene)	Benzodiazepine	60–100	Slow	7.5–22.5	Yes
Quazepam (Doral)	Benzodiazepine	50–200	Fast	7.5–15	Yes
Flurazepam (Dalmane)	Benzodiazepine	50–200	Fast	15–30	Yes

Note. ªNot available in the United States.

Adverse effects of benzodiazepine receptor agonists include daytime sedation, motor incoordination, slow reaction times, impaired memory function, confusional states, withdrawal states, rebound insomnia, respiratory depression, tolerance to drug effect, and potential for abuse.

Benzodiazepines do not stimulate the activity of hepatic microsomal enzyme systems, unlike many of the older hypnotic agents (e.g., barbiturates); thus, their long-term administration does not result in the accelerated metabolism of other pharmacological agents.

Benzodiazepines as a rule have prominent anxiolytic, muscle-relaxant, and anticonvulsant effects, as well as sedative-hypnotic effects. Normal doses of benzodiazepines given intermittently should be tolerated with minimal side effects (Bunney et al. 1999). Longer-half-life benzodiazepines, such as flurazepam, lorazepam, and clonazepam, can help maintain sleep longer as well as provide associated daytime antianxiety effect. A long-acting drug, such as clorazepate, may be ideal for patients with insomnia associated with anxiety.

Most benzodiazepines have similar effects on actual sleep quality and architecture. They tend to suppress or delay rapid eye movement sleep and increase the duration of Stage II sleep and may slightly decrease the amount of Stage III and Stage IV or deep sleep. The reduction in Stage III and Stage IV sleep induced by benzodiazepines leads to their occasional use as adjuncts in the treatment of Stage III and Stage IV parasomnias (e.g., night terrors, somnambulism).

Nonbenzodiazepine Hypnotics

Two nonbenzodiazepines are currently available, which promote sedation by their agonist effect at the $GABA_A$ benzodiazepine-1 receptor subunit. Zolpidem became available in 1992 and zaleplon in 1999.

Both zaleplon and zolpidem have become commonly prescribed. Zolpidem is an imidazopyridine hypnotic with specific benzodiazepine receptor agonist properties (Drover et al. 2000). At a therapeutic dose level, it does not appear to alter normal sleep patterns. It has the advantage of rapid onset of action, short duration of action, minimal risk of tolerance and addiction, and minimal rebound insomnia at cessation of use. Zolpidem appears to have a low likelihood of adversely affecting memory or motor coordination; this finding is possibly related to its receptor specificity. Open trials have shown that zolpidem maintains subjective benefits in insomnia for as long as 180 days (Kummer et al. 1993). Because zolpidem is a benzodiazepine receptor agonist, its effects can also be reversed by flumazenil (Wesensten et al. 1995).

Zaleplon is a pyrazolopyrimidine with selective benzodiazepine-1 receptor agonist properties. It appears to have unique benefits related to its ultra-short duration of action and half-life of approximately 1.1 hours. The drug has a very rapid absorption and onset of action, comparable with those of zolpidem (Wagner et al. 1998). Its clearance is so rapid that at 4 hours after administration, there is no evidence of impairment of memory or cognition. Therefore, zaleplon can be administered not only as a bedtime hypnotic but also in the middle of the night, as long as the patient has 4 hours between ingestion of zaleplon and rising time. This allows the patient with nocturnal awakenings to take medication only if he or she needs it, rather than prophylactically at bedtime to ward off potential nocturnal awakening. Zaleplon has also shown efficacy over the long term, with no risk of rebound insomnia.

Melatonin

Considerable attention has recently been given to melatonin as a possible hypnotic agent. Melatonin is a neurohormone that is the principal indolamine of the pineal gland and is produced under the control of the suprachiasmatic nucleus. Serotonin is converted to melatonin by two enzymatic steps in the pinealocyte. Normally, when light levels decrease at night, melatonin production is stimulated. The production of melatonin during dark periods decreases in humans as they age. Because this reduction parallels the decrease in quality and quantity of sleep in elderly individuals, it has been postulated that melatonin deficiency may contribute to this disruption. This establishes the elderly as an appropriate population in which to carefully assess the benefits of melatonin as a hypnotic. High doses of melatonin (3–100 mg) have been suggested as producing hypnotic effects, especially in elderly individuals (Haimov et al. 1995). However, lower doses have been less consistent in terms of hypnotic effect, and melatonin's popularity in health food stores and the lay press has a placebo effect. Melatonin has a half-life of only 20–30 minutes, so it is likely to have an impact only on sleep onset. Double-blind studies have been inconsistent, finding both efficacy and lack of efficacy of melatonin as a hypnotic (Mendelson 1997; Zhdanova et al. 1996). Melatonin appears to have an important influence on the regulation of circadian periodicity, as well as mild hypnotic properties. It may have benefit in treatment of jet lag, shift work maladaptation syndrome, non-24-hour sleep–wake cycles, and delayed sleep phase syndrome, as discussed in Chapter 3.

Melatonin as a therapeutic agent is not yet approved by the U.S. Food and Drug Administration. Thus, type of manufacture, relative purity, and accuracy of dose are not controlled. Adequate dose–response and toxicity studies have not yet been conducted. Melatonin has widespread effects on sexual behavior and reproduction in animals; the extent to which such effects may occur in humans is unknown. In addition, the potential of melatonin to worsen depression and even cause vasoconstriction has been suggested. Therefore, we must alert the reader to the fact that its safety and efficacy remain largely unknown. We suggest caution when recommending its long-term use, especially in children.

■ OVER-THE-COUNTER AND ALTERNATIVE PHARMACOLOGICAL TREATMENTS

Survey data suggest that between 20% and 40% of Americans use complementary or alternative therapies. Often these therapies are used for chronic conditions, including insomnia and fatigue. Although numerous compounds are widely used, the effects on sleep and alertness are unclear because of the lack of large, double-blind, randomized placebo-controlled studies. Currently, we cannot recommend the use of these agents and suggest that consumers be cautious about using (especially regularly or excessively) any over-the-counter agent.

Compounds that have been used as treatments for insomnia include valerian, kava, and passionflower. A number of studies of valerian have demonstrated a subjective decrease in sleep latency and time awake during the night after sleep onset. One small randomized study did demonstrate a slight increase in slow-wave sleep in patients with psychophysiological insomnia (Donath et al. 2000). Kava has been shown in a number of clinical trials to have some antianxiety effects, often similar to those of benzodiazepine medications. Passionflower is used as a sedative agent, but no studies of it alone could be found.

Ephedrine is used to improve alertness and decrease fatigue. It does have a central alerting effect, but this is less pronounced than the central alerting effect of amphetamine. The peripheral effects, especially on blood pressure and heart rate, appear to predominate and can lead to adverse, even fatal, outcomes.

■ TREATMENT OF CHRONIC INSOMNIA

Chronic insomnia is a challenging and often frustrating medical complaint for both patient and physician. Commonly, medical or psychiatric causes of insomnia can be treated successfully (see Chapter 3). However, a considerable group of patients who have primary insomnia or insomnia secondary to an underlying illness or to a problem related to age, chronic pain, drug therapy, or a chronic medical condition still require a strategy to provide regular or intermittent sedation for some degree of relief or comfort. One such plan is to prescribe a sedative-hypnotic one to four times per week, to reduce risk of habituation, maintain potency, and still provide intermittent sleep. This medication should be given in conjunction with strong efforts to reinforce good sleep hygiene and other behavioral techniques. Patients with chronic anxiety or chronic overstimulation by medication such as theophylline may function well with use of sedative-hypnotics.

Patients whose insomnia is related in part to chronic anxiety may respond better to a benzodiazepine than to zolpidem or zaleplon, because benzodiazepines have much greater anxiolytic effects. The clinician must therefore be cautious about habituation and dependence.

Chronic insomnias that are not related significantly to anxiety might be well managed with zolpidem or zaleplon, because the risk of tolerance, dependence, and abuse is minimal, and several studies support the safety and efficacy of long-term daily use (Greenblatt et al. 1998).

There may be a group of patients with chronic insomnia complaints—some of whom have other associated medical complaints and symptoms (e.g., chronic fatigue, chronic pain, and peripheral neuropathy)—whose complaints appear to be managed well with relatively low doses of sedating antidepressants. This includes depressed patients taking serotonin reuptake inhibitors whose sleep might benefit from adjunctive use of drugs such as trazodone or mirtazapine. Such groups are not yet clearly defined by specific pathophysiology, signs, or symptoms, however, and the necessary well-controlled studies showing efficacy are not generally available. Nonetheless, we suggest that agents such as those listed in Table 7–3 may be of help to these patients.

In addition, some patients with mood and anxiety disorders, posttraumatic stress disorder, or psychosis continue to have insomnia even after what appears to be adequate treatment of the illness. Also, patients with dementia may require medication to sleep and to reduce nocturnal agitation. Mood stabilizers, antipsychotics and other psychotropic medications listed in Table 7–4 may be of benefit as adjunctive or alternative treatments in these situations.

TABLE 7–3. **Antidepressant medications with sedative properties**

Drug	Dose (mg)	Uses/Advantages
Amitriptyline (Elavil)	10–100	Chronic pain, peripheral neuropathy, fibromyalgia
Doxepin (Sinequan)	10–200	Chronic fatigue syndrome, fibromyalgia, post–alcohol withdrawal insomnia, adjunct to nonsedating SSRIs
Trazodone (Desyrel)	25–400	Adjunct to nonsedating SSRIs (warn men about incidence of priapism and potential need for immediate withdrawal from drug; also, warn patients about orthostatic hypotension)
Nortriptyline (Pamelor)	10–100	Depression or anxiety disorder and insomnia, chronic pain
Nefazodone (Serzone)	100–600	Depression with anxiety (sedation is less than that of trazodone, without risk of orthostatic changes or priapism)
Mirtazapine (Remeron)	15–60	Serotonergic and noradrenergic mechanisms; somnolence and weight gain are common side effects

Note. SSRI=selective serotonin reuptake inhibitor.

TABLE 7–4. Medications with sedative-hypnotic properties used to treat insomnia

Drug	Dose (mg)	Uses
Mood stabilizers		
Carbamazepine (Tegretol)	100–800	PTSD, nightmares, night terrors, agitated drug withdrawal states
Gabapentin (Neurontin)	100–3,600	PTSD, nightmares, night terrors, agitated drug withdrawal states, chronic insomnia
Divalproex (Depakote)	125–2,000	PTSD, nightmares, night terrors, agitated drug withdrawal states
Oxcarbazepine (Trileptal)	150–2,400	PTSD, central nervous system overstimulation syndromes
Antipsychotics		
Chlorpromazine (Thorazine)	25–500	Generally restricted to patients with psychosis
Haloperidol (Haldol)	0.5–40	Occasionally effective for agitation and dementia
Quetiapine (Seroquel)	2.5–1,200	Psychosis, treatment-resistant insomnia, agitated states
Olanzapine (Zyprexa)	2.5–20	Psychosis, agitated states, mania
Risperidone (Risperdal)	0.25–6	Psychosis, agitation with dementia
Other agents		
Diphenhydramine (Benadryl)	25–100	Allergies, mild insomnia, patients at risk for medication abuse, patients taking antipsychotic medications with extrapyramidal side effects such as muscle dystonia or parkinsonian-like tremor
Cyproheptadine (Periactin)	4–40	PTSD, cluster headaches with insomnia
Buspirone (Buspar)	5–40	Occasionally effective for nocturnal agitation in elderly patients
Clonidine (Catapres)	0.1–1.2	Opiate withdrawal insomnia, refractory PTSD, treatment-resistant bipolar disorder, hot flashes or sweating

Note. PTSD=posttraumatic stress disorder.

■ REFERENCES

Bunney WE Jr, Azarnoff DL, Brown BW Jr, et al: Report of the Institute of Medicine Committee on the Efficacy and Safety of Halcion. Arch Gen Psychiatry 56:349–352, 1999

Donath F, Quispe S, Diefenbach K, et al: Critical evaluation of the effect of valerian extract on sleep structure and quality. Pharmacopsychiatry 33:47–53, 2000

Drover D, Lemmens H, Naidu S, et al: Pharmacokinetics, pharmacodynamics, and relative pharmacokinetic/pharmacodynamic profiles of zaleplon and zolpidem. Clin Ther 22:1443–1461, 2000

Greenblatt DJ, Harmatz JS, von Moltke LL, et al: Comparative kinetics and dynamics of zaleplon, zolpidem, and placebo. Clin Pharmacol Ther 64:553–561, 1998

Haimov I, Lavie P, Laudon M, et al: Melatonin replacement therapy of elderly insomniacs. Sleep 18:598–603, 1995

Kummer J, Guendel L, Eich FX, et al: Long-term polysomnographic study of the efficacy and safety of zolpidem in elderly psychiatric in-patients with insomnia. J Int Med Res 21:291–313, 1993

Mendelson WB: Efficacy of melatonin as a hypnotic agent. J Biol Rhythms 12:651–656, 1997

Mendelson WB, Jain B: An assessment of short-acting hypnotics. Drug Saf 13:247–270, 1995

Wagner J, Wagner ML, Hening WA: Beyond benzodiazepines: alternative pharmacologic agents for the treatment of insomnia. Ann Pharmacother 32:680–691, 1998

Wesensten NJ, Balkin TJ, Davis HQ, et al: Reversal of triazolam- and zolpidem-induced memory impairment by flumazenil. Psychopharmacology (Berl) 121:242–249, 1995

Zhdanova IV, Wurtman RJ, Morabito C, et al: Effects of low oral doses of melatonin, given 2–4 hours before habitual bedtime, on sleep in normal young humans. Sleep 19:423–431, 1996

■ RECOMMENDED READING

Hobbs WR, Rall TW, Verdoorn TA: Hypnotics and sedatives: ethanol, in Goodman and Gilman's The Pharmacological Basis of Therapeutics. Edited by Hardman JG, Limbird LE, Molinoff PB, et al. New York, McGraw-Hill, 1996, pp 361–398

8

SPECIAL PROBLEMS
AND POPULATIONS

■ SLEEP PROBLEMS IN CHILDREN

In this section, we address the most frequently encountered sleep problems in infants and children. Both symptomatic presentations and sleep disturbances that often accompany specific diagnostic categories in infants and children are included. Diagnosis and management of sleep disorders in children are similar to those of adult sleep disturbances: the clinician first must assess carefully whether a medical condition may be associated with the child's sleep complaint and, if so, treat this condition as appropriate. Children with developmental disabilities, blindness, and other medical disorders may have significant sleep difficulties that should be evaluated in the context of their disorders (Leger et al. 1999; Wiggs 2001).

Sleep Problems During Infancy and Early Childhood

Ferber (1987) made an important point about insomnia in infants and children:

> There is an important difference between the "insomnias" of the young child and that of the adult. An insomniac adult remains awake despite his own desires and efforts to fall asleep. A sleepless infant or toddler also remains awake, but in this case it is despite his parents' desires and efforts to have him fall asleep. "Insomnia" as experienced by adults probably does not occur before middle childhood (p. 141).

Most sleep problems in infancy result from either sleep disturbances, in somewhat atypical infants, or parental difficulties in handling potentially time-limited sleep disturbances that then become chronic disturbances of sleep habits.

Most infants entrain their circadian systems to a 24-hour sleep–wake rhythm ("settle") by age 16 weeks (range, 3–6 months). By then, they sleep fairly well throughout the night and are awake predominantly during the daytime hours. It is difficult to be certain that an infant younger than 6 months has a sleep problem because of normal variability in settling. Occasional nighttime awakenings are to be expected thereafter, but these need not require parental attention.

Sleep difficulties in the young infant are often associated either with excessive nighttime feeding or with unusual habits learned in association with sleep transition (Ferber 1987).

By age 6 months, infants can obtain adequate nutrition during daytime feedings, so they do not need nighttime feedings. Persistent nighttime feeding can lead both to expectations on the part of the infant (with habit-associated arousals or difficulty returning to sleep without feeding) and to arousals associated with excessive voiding and wet diapers as a result of the feedings. Eliminating these nighttime feedings can solve these problems.

Habits acquired in association with the transition from wakefulness to sleep can be a problem area. Infants who have an elaborate ritual associated with going to sleep may have difficulty returning to sleep after normal awakenings without a similar ritual. Infants who fall asleep outside their cribs (e.g., in a room with the lights, radio, or television on) and who are then moved to their cribs may not be able to return to sleep after awakenings without the same conditions being present. Similarly, if the child who awakens spontaneously is always removed from the crib and rocked, cradled, or carried, a habit pattern may ensue in which the infant cannot return to sleep in the absence of these conditions. A careful history will help elucidate such associations, which can then be corrected by the parents. Parents may require considerable support in these efforts because infants typically will initially resist the efforts to institute new sleep habits.

A child who has had disturbed sleep in conjunction with a developmental disorder (e.g., colic—discussed in the next paragraph), a medical illness, or a developmental delay in sleep consolidation may have developed, along with the parents, atypical habits associated with sleep onset or nighttime awakenings. Such habits and the associated sleep disruption can persist, even after the initial developmental problem or other problem is resolved. Thus, although it may be informative to examine conditions surrounding the onset of a sleep complaint, the persistence of the complaint may be related more to ongoing poor sleep habits than to the initial problem itself, which may well have been resolved. Treatment should be directed toward the poor sleep habits.

Colic in infancy can pose special problems, and because it may affect one in four infants, it deserves mention (Weissbluth 1987). Colic is characterized by unexplained paroxysms of crying, fussing, irritability, increased motor tone, and wakefulness. Colic usually begins during the first several weeks of age, lasts for several months, and dissipates by age 4 months. Its etiology is unclear, but colic may represent normally maturing physiological processes rather than a deficiency or developmental delay in central nervous system inhibitory mechanisms, as was formerly suspected. Sleep disturbances are common and difficult to treat in infants with colic, but these problems should begin to resolve by age 4 months. If they do not resolve by this age, the parents may not have established a sufficiently regular sleep–wake schedule. This lack of a regular schedule is perhaps a result of their initial experience with their infant and suggests that the infant could not adapt to the schedule anyway. This problem probably would have been undeniable during the first 4 months but may no longer be true. Thus, the parents' experience during the initial 4 months may shape their parenting style in a manner that is subsequently inappropriate for encouraging regular sleep–wake behavior in their infant.

Sleep Problems During Middle Childhood

During the latency period (approximately ages 4–12 years), sleep is generally good, and few children have complaints. Parasomnias (e.g., night terrors, sleepwalking) are not infrequent during this period, however, and a careful history of unusual nocturnal behaviors will suggest their presence (see Chapter 5). Problems that do occur during this period are usually associated with difficulty convincing the child to go to sleep and can often be traced to poor limit setting. A consistent bedtime ritual consonant with good sleep hygiene (regular bedtime and arousal time, quiet and darkened sleeping room, no distractions) will help alleviate such problems. Children are, of course, also susceptible to sleep disturbance caused by daytime stress factors. Parental concern and reassurance, as well as allowing the child to talk about difficulties, may be helpful. Occasional transient insomnias—for example, a night when the child says that he or she cannot fall asleep because of worry about not being able to sleep—can be alleviated by suggesting that the child think about a recent pleasurable experience rather than thinking about going to sleep. Sleep will often follow. The child with severe nighttime fears and unusual fearfulness during the day may present a special problem, and special counseling may be required.

Primary snoring occurs in as many as 1 in 10 children and may not require specific treatment. It must, however, be distinguished from snoring secondary to obstructive sleep apnea, which does require treatment (Carroll and Loughlin 1995). Obstructive sleep apnea in children is usually caused by adenotonsillar hypertrophy and generally is successfully treated by tonsillectomy and adenoidectomy (Davidson-Ward and Marcus 1996).

Sleep Problems During Adolescence

Adolescents undergo major developmental changes, experience multiple changes in their own roles and in roles expected of them, and enter a period when other disorders affecting sleep (e.g., narcolepsy, depression) may emerge. Thus, stress- and schedule-related insomnia is more common among adolescents than in younger children. Poor sleep hygiene is often a prominent etiological factor in disturbed sleep; this condition sometimes masquerades as a delayed sleep phase–like syndrome. Initial screening of adolescents with insomnia complaints should emphasize sleep habits and sleep schedule, social- and school-related stress factors, family difficulties, drug and alcohol use, and possible emergence of other medical (e.g., narcolepsy) or psychiatric (e.g., depression) disorders. Any disturbances should be evaluated carefully to determine if and how they relate to the sleep complaint. Recent studies have demonstrated a strong link between onset of sleep problems in adolescents and both depression and cigarette smoking (Patten et al. 2000).

Major psychiatric disorders may emerge during adolescence. Evidence of disturbed thinking, paranoid ideation, hypomania, or grandiosity or marked difficulties in school should alert the clinician to the possibility of a psychiatric disorder. The emergence of schizophrenia may be heralded by frequent terrifying nightmares and associated insomnia.

Excessive daytime sleepiness (EDS) may be associated with the onset of narcolepsy, which often first presents as falling asleep in school. A common cause of EDS in adolescents is depression, which occurs more frequently than in adults.

Treatment of sleep complaints in adolescents is appropriately directed initially at an underlying primary disorder. Insomnias related to stress and poor sleep hygiene respond well to behavioral techniques, including enforcement of regular schedules, education about good sleep hygiene, sleep restriction, and relaxation or biofeedback training. Counseling may be indicated to resolve family disturbances. Pharmacological agents should probably not be included in the first line of treatment, unless, of course, they are indicated for an underlying problem such as depression.

Circadian Schedule Disorders in Children

Infants, latency-age children, and adolescents all are susceptible to circadian rhythm–based sleep disorders such as delayed sleep phase syndrome (DSPS) (Ferber 1987). Some evidence suggests that adolescents may have a physiological delay in circadian rhythms, which may, in part, explain their tendency to stay up very late and then try to sleep late in the morning. The tendency to develop these disorders likely has a familial component, which, when compounded by family practices that reinforce staying up late and sleeping in the morning, can result in quite profound sleep disturbances. The clinician should keep in mind the association between DSPS and depression in adolescents (Thorpy et al. 1988).

DSPS may begin to cause difficulties when children start school and when regular early-morning awakening becomes important. However, DSPS more often first appears in adolescence. The parents often must struggle to convince the adolescent to go to sleep at night, and they may then have equal difficulty awakening him or her in the morning. These adolescents tend to sleep late on weekends to recoup sleep lost during the week. A careful history and sleep diary will facilitate diagnosis. There may be a family history of similar problems. Treatment consists of a regular sleep schedule for both weekdays and weekends, with a regular bedtime and a regular, early arousal time. Treatment with morning bright light exposure, as used for adult DSPS, may prove efficacious in adolescents, and evening melatonin has also been reported to help in DSPS (Dahlitz et al. 1991).

Children who are blind or mentally retarded or who have organic central nervous system disturbances can have quite profound circadian schedule disturbances, which frequently manifest as sleep disorders. Such children may develop free-running non-24-hour sleep–wake rhythms that can be quite disruptive. Melatonin (0.5 mg at bedtime) has been described as useful in entraining free-running circadian rhythms in a child (Lapierre and Dumont 1995). Melatonin has also been reported as being helpful in children with selected developmental disorders (Jan 2000), but the safety and efficacy of long-term melatonin use in children are not yet known.

Attention-Deficit/Hyperactivity Disorder

Children with attention-deficit/hyperactivity disorder (ADHD) frequently have disturbed sleep, including difficulty falling asleep, restless sleep, and early-morning awakening (Owens et al. 2000). Despite sleep-related complaints in children with ADHD, little polysomnographic evidence exists to support a particular type of sleep disturbance that accompanies ADHD (Corkum et al. 1999). Actigraphic studies support the concept of instability of sleep patterns in ADHD (Gruber et al. 2000). Although routine polysomnograms (PSGs) are not indicated in ADHD, careful sleep histories should be obtained from all such children to avoid missing a bona fide sleep disorder such as sleep apnea or periodic limb movement disorder (PLMD), which should be treated and may contribute to the ADHD symptom profile (Owens et al. 2000; Picchietti et al. 1998).

Medications used to treat ADHD include stimulants such as methylphenidate and dextroamphetamine, which are known to alter sleep patterns, as well as monoamine oxidase inhibitors (MAOIs) and tricyclics, which are known to suppress rapid eye movement (REM) sleep. Indeed, many of the sleep problems seen in ADHD might be related to either 1) pharmacotherapy for ADHD or 2) comorbid conditions, such as depression (Mick et al. 2000). Methylphenidate treatment of ADHD in children has been shown to delay sleep onset, lengthen sleep time, and normalize certain REM sleep parameters. Dextroamphetamine treatment of ADHD may result in delayed sleep onset, decreased sleep efficiency, increased REM sleep latency, and decreased REM sleep time. However, these medication-induced changes also may be associated with diminished nocturnal arousals and improved overall sleep. The clinician should remember that symptoms of inadequate nocturnal sleep—such as inattention, irritability, distractibility, and impulsivity—can resemble symptoms of ADHD (Dahl 1995).

Sleep Laboratory Studies in Infants and in Children

A polysomnographic recording usually is not indicated for most sleep problems in children, especially if a careful clinical evaluation strongly suggests an insomnia possibly related to stress, schedule, or poor hygiene. It is perhaps more reasonable to begin with a good clinical evaluation and then to assess clinical response to treatment; polysomnography should be reserved for problems that do not respond to treatment. In this age group, polysomnographic studies are not particularly helpful in the case of sleep complaints associated with psychiatric disorders. The clinician who is evaluating EDS should use a PSG and, in most cases, a Multiple Sleep Latency Test (MSLT). Assessment of daytime sleepiness in childhood may include strategies above and beyond a single MSLT, such as actigraphy and assessment of cognitive function (Kotagal and Goulding 1996). Restless leg syndrome and PLMD may be seen in children, and the latter may complicate ADHD. A PSG may be indicated in such cases.

■ ENURESIS

Presenting Complaints

- Wetting the bed at night—evident usually in children
- Frequent urination during the day
- Feelings of guilt or shame

Clinical Presentation

Most individuals with enuresis have *primary enuresis*—that is, they have never had a consistently dry period. In these patients, nighttime bed-wetting, which is expected of an infant or a young child, persists well past the time of normal toilet training. Although there is no strict agreement by clinicians, most believe that enuresis that occurs after age 5 years deserves evaluation and treatment. These patients often have a need to urinate frequently during the day. Occasional daytime "accidents" also may occur. The patients may awaken during the night after wetting the bed or may not notice the fact until morning. The enuretic child frequently feels guilty and ashamed about his or her nighttime accidents. The child's social activity may be restricted because he or she is embarrassed to participate in activities outside the home, such as sleeping at friends' houses, visiting relatives, and camping. *Secondary enuresis* is enuresis that has started after the individual has had dry nighttime periods for at least 3 months.

Incidence

In the general population, 15% of boys and 10% of girls are estimated to have enuresis at age 5 years. Approximately 5%–10% of enuretic patients have secondary enuresis (Nino-Murcia and Keenan 1987).

Etiology and Pathophysiology

The vast majority of enuretic children have no discernible urinary tract dysfunction, especially if they do not have symptoms such as urgency, abnormalities in stream or flow, or daytime enuresis. Most enuretic children have a small functional bladder capacity, which may be considered a maturational delay of bladder development. Some studies have suggested that enuretic children have more and stronger bladder contractions than do nonenuretic children. The bladder of the enuretic child can be thought of as one that fills quickly, contracts vigorously, and faces little resistance. Secondary enuresis raises the index of suspicion that an organic problem may be involved or that the enuresis is in response to a stressful situation or a conflict. Anatomical conditions that are uncommonly associated with enuresis include a congenitally small bladder, wide bladder neck anomalies, bladder outflow obstruction, urethral diverticula, ectopic ureters, and epispadias. Medical conditions such as urinary tract infections, diabetes mellitus, and diabetes insipidus also are associated with enuresis. Occasionally, enuresis is a concurrent symptom of obstructive sleep apnea.

Laboratory Findings

Laboratory studies have demonstrated that the sleep of enuretic children is normal. Because enuresis occurs during all stages of sleep, sleep laboratory studies are not thought to be indicated in most enuretic children.

Differential Diagnosis

A history of continuing enuresis with no intervening dry periods, especially with a positive family history, strongly suggests primary enuresis. Abnormalities of flow and/or urgency or the presence of other symptoms raises the index of suspicion for other medical etiologies. Nocturnal seizures with urinary incontinence should be differentiated from simple enuresis. Patients with nocturnal epilepsy often have histories of diurnal seizures as well. Vigorous motor activity or tongue biting during sleep may be evident. A clinical daytime electroencephalogram or expanded PSG is occasionally needed to determine whether nocturnal seizures are the cause of the enuresis.

Treatment

Most clinicians use a standard treatment plan for enuresis (Tobias 2000). A flowchart for the treatment of enuresis is shown in Figure 8–1.

Step 1: Initial evaluation.   The initial evaluation should include a thorough medical and sleep history (especially with respect to symptoms of diabetes mellitus, seizures, snoring, or a urinary tract infection) and a complete physical examination. The clinician should obtain and review a 2-week data log used to record times of meals (snacks included), the number of bathroom trips (both daytime and nighttime), hours of sleep, and bed-wetting incidents. The clinician should examine a urine sample for glycosuria or signs of infection. Urine volume should be measured to estimate the functional bladder capacity. The amount of urine voided can be determined at home by the parent or child, using a measuring cup. The guideline is that children ages 6–12 years have a bladder capacity of about 1 oz per year of age. If the clinician detects abnormalities on physical examination or by urinalysis, he or she should further evaluate the patient or seek specialty consultation.

Step 2: Discussion of the nature of enuresis and the treatment plan with the patient and his or her parents.   A system of rewards to be given to the child for dry nights should be established. The clinician should encourage the child's participation by asking the child to state why he or she wants to overcome the enuresis.

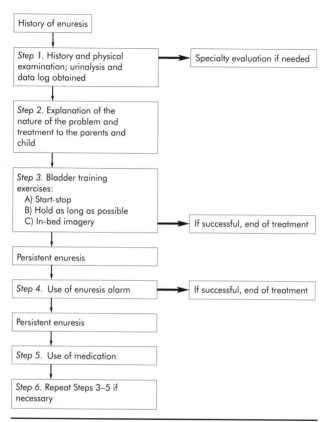

FIGURE 8–1. **Flowchart for treatment of enuresis.**

Often, asking the child to change his or her pajamas or bedclothes relieves the guilt that the child feels of having a parent clean up after him or her.

Step 3: Bladder training exercises. The clinician may ask the child to do a "start and stop" exercise (5–10 times per micturition) every time he or she urinates. This exercise may strengthen the external sphincter and give the child the sensation of controlling urination.

In another exercise, the child is given a large amount of his or her favorite liquid to drink twice a week. The child then attempts to retain the urine as long as possible before voiding. Weekly measurements of the amount voided should be recorded to observe whether the functional bladder capacity is increasing.

In yet another exercise, the child lies in bed after he or she has consumed a large quantity of liquid. The child pretends to be asleep and practices holding his or her urine until he or she gets up and goes to the bathroom.

Often these bladder training exercises alone increase the functional bladder capacity, decrease the number of bathroom trips during the day, and terminate the enuresis.

Step 4: Enuresis alarm.　If the child's enuresis persists after a few weeks of bladder training exercises, an enuresis alarm can be used. The most effective alarms are those that are triggered by a small amount of urine, with the sensor located in the underwear. The alarm should be positioned close to the child's ear (the alarm is usually clipped to the shirt collar). The child must get up and go to the bathroom when he or she is awakened by the alarm. The combination of bladder training exercises and an enuresis alarm is very effective in treating primary enuresis.

Step 5: Medication.　The clinician may consider administering medication if, as is occasionally the case, enuresis persists after bladder training exercises and an alarm have been used. Imipramine (25–50 mg 30 minutes before bedtime) has been commonly prescribed in the past, but its mechanism of action is not known. Desmopressin acetate (starting at 20 mg) via nasal spray has been shown to be effective, although relapses after cessation of therapy are common (Mark and Frank 1995).

Step 6: Repeat Steps 3–5.　If the child has a relapse after initial success, steps 3 through 5 should be repeated.

■ SLEEP IN ELDERLY INDIVIDUALS

Presenting Complaints

Elderly patients have increased sleep complaints and objectively measured sleep abnormalities. Presenting complaints often include

- Difficulty falling asleep and staying asleep
- Early-morning awakening, with difficulty returning to sleep
- Unrefreshing sleep
- Excessive tiredness or fatigue during the day
- Unusual behaviors during the sleep period
- Unusual nocturnal behaviors

Clinical Presentation

Most of the sleep problems seen in younger adults may also affect elderly adults; in addition, problems unique to or more frequent in elderly people exist. Proper clinical evaluation and treatment are very important in elderly patients; the clinician must not pass off sleep complaints as a "normal" part of aging or reflexively prescribe a hypnotic medication without first properly evaluating the complaint. Although many elderly patients complain primarily about their sleep problems, some need to be questioned directly about such issues because they may consider them a normal part of getting older and thus not worth mentioning. Frequently, family members (when elderly persons are living at home) or nursing staff (when elderly persons are in hospitals or nursing homes) will report unusual sleep habits or behaviors in elderly patients. The clinician must listen carefully to such complaints because they may contain important clues to etiology.

Incidence

The incidence of insomnia complaints increases dramatically in the elderly population. Estimates vary, but one study in the Los Angeles area found that 48% of those older than 50 years had insomnia (Bixler et al. 1979). A study involving 9,000 individuals age 65 or older found that only 20% rarely or never had sleep complaints. Between 23% and 34% had insomnia complaints, and 7%–15% rarely or never felt rested in the morning (Foley et al. 1995). Several, but not all, studies have found substantial increases in both sleep apnea and PLMD in asymptomatic, otherwise healthy elderly individuals. The range of increase varies considerably, however—up to 20%–30% or more of the elderly population. It is not yet clear whether the increase in these disorders is a normal part of the aging process (Ancoli-Israel et al. 1987; Mosko et al. 1988; Reynolds et al. 1985).

Etiology and Pathophysiology

The etiology of sleep complaints in elderly patients can be attributed to several mechanisms:

- The aging process may be associated with normal alterations in physiological systems controlling sleep and sleep behaviors.
- Specific sleep disorders, such as PLMD, sleep apnea, and REM sleep behavior disorder, appear to have an increased incidence with age.
- Psychiatric and medical disorders that adversely affect sleep have an increased incidence with age.
- Elderly people frequently take a variety of medications, for a variety of reasons, that may either interact or act differently in elderly individuals and result in altered sleep patterns or sleep behavior.
- Elderly persons are at high risk for economic stress, loss, and bereavement, all of which negatively affect sleep.

Sleep electroencephalogram morphology changes with age: Stage III and Stage IV sleep diminish in amount, and Stage I and Stage II sleep increase in proportion. Wakefulness, the number of arousals, and sleep fragmentation increase with age. Some of the apparent decrease in Stage III and Stage IV sleep may be related to the generally poorer level of aerobic fitness in older persons (Foley et al. 1995). These changes may be associated with a perceived lessened quality and/or quantity of sleep. Increased arousals and consequent sleep fragmentation result in an increased level of daytime sleepiness. Some studies have demonstrated a slight decrease in the amount of REM sleep.

The neurobiological systems that control the timing of circadian biorhythms, including the sleep–wake cycle, may become less efficient with age and less able to adapt to change. Evidence indicates a dampened circadian rest–activity rhythm with advancing age and a similarly dampened circadian body temperature rhythm. In elderly individuals, nocturnal melatonin secretion has been shown to be diminished (Haimov et al. 1995), which possibly contributes to both increased body temperature and poorer sleep. Thus, circadian schedules in elderly individuals may be more susceptible to interruptions. This possible increased susceptibility is especially important in patients in nursing homes, where clear day–night differences in light, noise, and activity may be diminished. Also, decreased growth hormone secretion associated with decreased amounts of slow-wave sleep, as well as a possible increase in resting plasma norepinephrine and cortisol levels (Van Cauter et al. 2000), is evident in elderly individuals. The latter finding could be related to both the sleep fragmentation and the decreased amount of REM sleep noted in elderly individuals.

The increase in PLMD and restless legs syndrome that occurs with aging may affect sleep quality, usually resulting in what is perceived as insomnia. The increased frequency of sleep apnea is not necessarily associated with hemodynamic or cardiovascular consequences, although it may be associated with increased daytime sleepiness.

Psychiatric disorders—especially depression, including bereavement-related depression—increase in frequency with increased age; in addition, the sleep disturbances associated with these disorders, such as early-morning awakening, are more common. Medical disorders—particularly those associated with chronic pain (e.g., osteoarthritis)—are more frequent and interfere with sleep in elderly persons. Nocturia may aggravate an otherwise unapparent problem with falling back to sleep. Often the medications used to control medical symptoms aggravate sleep further. It is very important to consider the role of medications in inducing sleep problems in elderly patients. Studies have estimated that 10% of the elderly population in the United States consumes one-quarter of prescribed drugs. Prescription and nonprescription drugs that are frequently used by elderly patients and that may induce sleep problems are listed in Table 8–1. As hypnotic use increases in the elderly population, the ability to metabolize hypnotics may diminish, especially when renal or hepatic disease is present. Thus, a single dose may act longer and have a greater effect.

Laboratory Findings

Polysomnographic studies of nocturnal sleep in healthy elderly individuals have shown decreased sleep efficiency, an increased number of awakenings and total time awake (especially in the last 2 hours of the night), and markedly diminished Stage III and Stage IV sleep. These changes, which usually begin at about age 50 years, are age related and are generally more pronounced in men.

TABLE 8–1. **Prescription and nonprescription drugs that may induce sleep problems in elderly patients**

Alcohol

Antiarrhythmic agents

Caffeine

Methysergide

Nasal decongestants

Nicotine

Scopolamine agents

Some antihypertensives

Steroids

Stimulants

Thyroid hormone

Xanthine derivatives

Before considering a PSG, the clinician must assess other possible causes of the complaint. He or she must evaluate medical conditions and treatment efficacy, may need to change medications or reduce doses, and should attempt to improve sleep hygiene and sleep schedules. Then, if the clinician strongly suspects the presence of specific abnormalities (such as apnea, PLMD, or REM sleep behavior disorder) that require a PSG for confirmation, he or she should consider the use of a sleep laboratory.

Polysomnographic interpretation in elderly patients is complicated by both the sleep-disrupting effects of concurrent illness and the medications used in this age group. If a PSG is obtained, shortened REM sleep latency may suggest an affective disorder component to a sleep complaint. The PSG may also help to separate early dementia (normal REM sleep latency) from depression (shortened REM sleep latency). REM sleep behavior disorder can be documented by characteristic increases in electromyographic activity during REM sleep.

Differential Diagnosis

The differential diagnosis of sleep complaints in elderly patients is one of the most demanding tasks in sleep disorders medicine. Rigor, thoroughness, and a high index of suspicion are necessary. A decision tree similar to that proposed for the differential diagnosis of chronic insomnia (see Figure 3–1 in Chapter 3) is appropriate, and the clinician must pay special attention to, and systematically explore, the following issues:

- Have poor sleep habits (e.g., spending excessive time in bed, keeping the radio or television on, taking excessive daytime naps, and not exercising) contributed to the complaint?
- Does the patient live in a stressful situation, or has he or she experienced a significant loss (e.g., death of a loved one)?
- Have coexisting medical disorders been adequately evaluated and optimally treated? Might some be unrecognized? Could treatment of these disorders be interfering with sleep?

- To what extent are medications (prescription or otherwise), sedative-hypnotics, alcohol, caffeine, and nicotine contributing to the complaint? (A trial reduction of doses or elimination of all but clearly medically necessary drugs is often helpful in differential diagnosis.)
- Is unrecognized depression or dementia playing a role in the sleep complaint?

Excessive nocturnal movements, especially when accompanied by dream mentation, should increase suspicion for a possible REM sleep behavior disorder, which is much more common in elderly men. The differential diagnosis also includes other parasomnias (e.g., somnambulism, night terrors) and nocturnal seizure disorder.

Treatment

Treatments of sleep complaints in elderly patients include those specific to identified pathophysiologies, such as concurrent medical illness, pain, PLMD, and depression, as well as an emphasis on behavioral strategies (Morin et al. 1999; Prinz 1995). Strict attention to good sleep hygiene is important, including not spending excessive time in bed and improving aerobic fitness if possible. Excessive use of caffeine, including that contained in over-the-counter analgesics, should be curtailed.

In elderly patients, bright light treatment has been useful in treating sleep disorders, including morning bright light for certain cases of sleep-onset insomnia (possibly caused by a mild circadian phase delay). Evening bright light has been found to be effective in sleep-maintenance insomnia in healthy elderly subjects (Campbell et al. 1995).

REM sleep behavior disorder may be effectively treated with clonazepam (0.5–1.0 mg at bedtime) in most patients.

Patients who are seen by several specialists and receive one or more prescriptions from each pose special problems. Ideally, one physician should manage all medications. The role of pharmacological agents must be tempered by the fact that half-lives may be extended, the possibility of multiple drug interactions is increased, and lower-than-usual doses may be adequate. The use of short-acting hypnotics such as zolpidem (5 mg) or zaleplon (5–10 mg) may be preferred to that of agents with longer half lives. Because relatively mild apnea in elderly patients infrequently has significant physiological consequences, the clinician must consider therapeutic intervention on an individual basis.

Treating sleep disturbances caused by dementia in elderly patients is an especially demanding task. A thorough medical evaluation to assess for occult infection, hypoxemia, urinary retention, and medication side effects and toxicity is a requisite first step. Behavioral issues may be important. Patients should try to increase daytime activity and light exposure while limiting (or eliminating) daytime napping. For patients with nocturnal agitation, drug therapy is generally necessary. The newer antipsychotic agents such as quetiapine or risperidone may be helpful; these drugs have fewer of the long-term effects associated with the antipsychotic agents historically used, such as thioridazine or haloperidol.

■ SLEEP PROBLEMS DURING PREGNANCY

Presenting Complaints

- Excessive sleepiness early in pregnancy
- Leg cramps
- Frightening dreams
- Difficulty falling asleep or staying asleep, usually beginning in the second or third trimester
- Backaches and/or physical discomfort interfering with sleep

Clinical Presentation

The first few weeks of pregnancy are often accompanied by complaints of increased sleep need and daytime sleepiness. Often these symptoms accompany nausea and morning sickness in early pregnancy. Sleep complaints are probably the rule rather than the exception by the third trimester, but the primary complaint during that time tends to be insomnia, either difficulty falling asleep, frequent awakening, or both. Sleep complaints secondary to non-pregnancy-related causes of disturbed sleep or insomnia may complicate the picture as well. Thus the clinician should maintain a high index of suspicion for disorders such as depression and anxiety.

Incidence

Up to two-thirds of pregnant women consider their sleep to be abnormal. Complaints include physical discomfort and backaches, awakenings typically described as "just waking up," increased urinary frequency, awakenings from fetal movements, heartburn, cramps or tingling in the legs, and difficulty falling asleep (Schweiger 1972). About 75% of these complaints appear to be related to the anatomical and physiological changes associated with pregnancy, but about 25% of the complaints are seemingly unrelated to the size of the uterus.

Etiology and Pathophysiology

The hormone progesterone may be connected to the excessive sleepiness in early pregnancy; a metabolite of progesterone has been found to act as a barbiturate-like ligand on the γ-aminobutyric acid receptor in the brain. The excessive sleepiness usually resolves spontaneously. Most sleep complaints later in pregnancy (especially in the third trimester) stem from the anatomical and physiological changes induced by the growing fetus. It is clear that as pregnancy progresses, it becomes increasingly difficult to find a comfortable sleeping position. The weight of the fetus and the enlarged uterus pressing on surrounding structures cause discomfort. The woman can no longer sleep on her stomach, and sleeping on her back or side is uncomfortable. As the fetus's head begins to press on the bladder, more frequent trips to the bathroom are likely. Not infrequently, a type of primary insomnia of pregnancy develops as well, but the pathophysiology of this insomnia is not yet understood.

The clinician must keep in mind that nothing prevents a pregnant woman from having other causes of disordered sleep, such as an affective or anxiety disorder, a circadian rhythm–based disorder, or PLMD. Women with histories of depression or anxiety who have stopped taking antidepressants or antianxiety agents in preparation for pregnancy or because of becoming pregnant have been shown to have very high rates of relapse (Altshuler et al. 2001). One study has suggested that 75% of women who stop antidepressant therapy relapse during pregnancy, and 59% of these women do so during the first trimester (Cohen 2000). This group often has sleep disturbance as an early symptom of relapse, or at least a prominent part of affective or anxiety relapse. Relapse risk should be carefully balanced against risk of fetal exposure to psychotropics during early pregnancy (Altshuler et al. 1996).

Laboratory Findings

During the third trimester, pregnant women have increased wake time after sleep onset, decreased sleep efficiency, decreased REM sleep, and increased Stage I sleep (Hertz et al. 1992). Diagnostic polysomnography is rarely required during pregnancy. A PSG would be necessary primarily for differential diagnosis of other suspected medical causes of the sleep complaint (e.g., narcolepsy, PLMD, sleep-related breathing disorder). In such cases, standard diagnostic criteria would generally apply.

Differential Diagnosis

Accurate differential diagnosis of pregnancy-related sleep complaints begins with a recognition of the "normal" sleep complaints during pregnancy and an evaluation of whether the patient's complaints differ from the normal ones. A detailed sleep history is important. Questions to be answered might include the following: Did the symptoms arise during the pregnancy, or did they antedate or become aggravated by the pregnancy? Is there reason to believe that the patient may have a concurrent sleep disorder unrelated to the pregnancy? The clinician must ask about early-morning awakenings (affective disorder), the duration of the complaint (whether it antedates pregnancy), and a possible association with stress or loss. He or she should note acute or gradual onset and whether the problem improves when the patient is away from home or the normal sleep environment (psychophysiological insomnia). Snoring, breathing pauses, excessive movement, shortness of breath or palpitations on awakening, and morning headaches may indicate disorders that would be best diagnosed by use of a nocturnal PSG. Evidence of chronic anxiety, panic attacks, or depression, including vegetative signs, would imply an anxiety or depressive disorder, which may require a psychiatric consultation.

Special pregnancy-related anxieties may relate to the feeling of being out of control of one's physiology. The pregnant woman begins to lose her usual figure, is susceptible to increased mood changes, is plagued at times by nausea and vomiting, is unable to sleep, and is discouraged from using customary medications that may help her sleep. She may also have concerns about being a good mother and fears about how her partner will react to the infant. She may be afforded no comfort from well-meaning friends who regale her with horror stories about how their children did not sleep through the night until they were 2 years old.

Treatment

The treatment of sleep complaints during pregnancy is complicated by the fact that most pharmacological medications should be used with great care and caution. The use of sleep hygiene and other behavioral techniques should be emphasized whenever possible. Of course, the clinician must recognize when a sleep complaint may be symptomatic of a more serious underlying disorder (e.g., major affective disorder). In these cases, psychotherapy is essential. In severe cases, pharmacological intervention may be necessary, as discussed later this chapter.

The most important aspect of treatment is, again, proper assessment and accurate diagnosis. If the sleep complaints fall within the "normal" range, education and reassurance that sleep will improve after delivery are helpful. Seeing a light at the end of the tunnel can be most encouraging.

The sleep position problems during the third trimester can often be best handled by judicious use of extra pillows. Evening fluid intake can be decreased. Customary sleep hygiene techniques should be emphasized (see Chapter 3).

The father plays a special role in the management of sleep disorders in pregnancy. He can help his pregnant partner with insomnia by providing support, by being available to her, and by helping her reduce some of the pressures resulting from her impaired daytime functioning. He may feel alienated by his partner's preoccupation with the unborn child and her impending relationship with the new child. It is important that the father not view his partner's insomnia-related fatigue as additional rejection or as evidence of emotional distancing. Appropriate counseling by the perceptive physician may be helpful in this regard. If the sleep problem is the result of a psychiatric disturbance or a primary sleep disorder requiring medication, the father must be involved in making decisions about medication use. The physician should explain potential hazards and inform both partners that medication is frequently a last resort.

At times, the pregnant woman may complain that her sleep is disturbed by her partner's disruptive sleep patterns or snoring. In such cases, appropriate evaluation of the father's sleep may be in order. Sleep problems seemingly independent of or in addition to those associated with pregnancy per se require special attention. Sleep restriction, relaxation, and perhaps even biofeedback may be appropriate when a significant psychophysiological insomnia component is likely present.

Pharmacological agents. Because there is no ethical way to systematically study pharmacological agents for safety in pregnancy, we are forced to rely on animal studies, anecdotal reports, and registries of retrospective experience with women taking various agents. We are clearly aware that alcohol use is highly contraindicated in pregnancy because of the risk of fetal alcohol syndrome or other adverse effects. Almost all sedative-hypnotics are either totally or relatively contraindicated because of potential teratogenicity. Pregnant women are typically recommended to stay clear of drugs in general, especially in the first trimester of pregnancy, to avoid increasing the risk of organ damage, withdrawal syndromes (in the case of use of medication in the third trimester), and behavioral problems (in the child in later years).

Patients with milder cases of insomnia with no obvious mood or anxiety disorder may benefit from eating food high in tryptophan, a serotonin precursor (e.g., bananas, milk, and some bakery products). More severe cases are very likely to represent mood and anxiety disorders.

Recent expert consensus is that pregnant women with severe mood and anxiety disorders should be given first-line treatment with serotonin reuptake inhibitors (SRIs), combined with cognitive or interpersonal psychotherapy. Relatively extensive experience with fluoxetine and sertraline in pregnancy shows no pattern of increased physical or behavioral abnormality. Choices of second-line agents would be other SRIs or tricyclic antidepressants. If insomnia persists after SRI treatment, alternative SRIs may be tried, or adjunctive use of a tricyclic agent such as amitriptyline or nortriptyline would be acceptable. A number of studies support the safety of tricyclics during pregnancy. The high risk of postpartum depression in pregnant women with histories of depression makes it usually unwise to try to taper medications before delivery. There have been some anecdotal reports suggesting early behavioral problems, such as increased irritability, feeding problems, and disrupted sleep in infants born with serum levels of SRIs, tricyclics, or benzodiazepines.

The only sedative-hypnotics currently considered acceptable for use during pregnancy are lorazepam and clonazepam. Historically, research suggested an increased frequency of cleft palate in children born to mothers taking benzodiazepines, but this finding has been questioned. If possible, benzodiazepines should still be tapered before delivery, to prevent infant irritability or feeding problems. The consensus regarding treatment of psychosis is to use high-potency neuroleptics such as haloperidol or, possibly, olanzapine (Goldstein et al. 2000). Electroconvulsive therapy is considered appropriate during pregnancy or the postpartum period for treatment-resistant cases or psychotic mood disorders.

There is some support of the use of verapamil in pregnant women with anxiety or bipolar disorders: verapamil has been used to treat fetal supraventricular tachycardias with no associated risk of teratogenicity.

Women with mild to moderate depression who find themselves pregnant while taking antidepressants are encouraged to gradually stop taking medication over 1–2 weeks or to switch to a "safer" SRI if risk of recurrent severe depression is too high.

During breast-feeding, of course, it is preferred that mothers take no medication, because virtually all medications end up in some concentration in breast milk. The first-line antidepressants to use during breast-feeding are, in order of preference, sertraline, fluoxetine or paroxetine, and tricyclics (Wisner et al. 1998). If it is essential that a patient take a sedative-hypnotic during breast-feeding, lorazepam is the recommended agent.

Sleep After Delivery

Physicians can reassure pregnant women that their sleep will likely improve rapidly after delivery, and this is usually the case, assuming other causes of a sleep disorder are not present. This fact alone will often be of substantial benefit to the patient with a pregnancy-related sleep complaint. However, the infant likely will be another source of disturbed sleep until he or she learns that it is appropriate to sleep at night and be active during the day. It is helpful to tell the mother what to expect in this regard. Sleep studies have shown a significant reduction in wake time after sleep onset and increased sleep efficiency 3–5 months postpartum, although the percentage of REM sleep remains low (Hertz et al. 1992).

■ SLEEP COMPLAINTS ASSOCIATED WITH PREMENSTRUAL SYNDROME

Presenting Complaints

- Insomnia or hypersomnia during specific times in the menstrual period
- Sleepwalking (parasomnias) during the premenstrual period
- Insomnia associated with premenstrual syndrome (PMS)

Clinical Presentation

Many women complain of difficulty sleeping or excessive sleepiness for several days during normal menstruation. Women with PMS often have prominent associated sleep complaints, usually of an insomnia type. In addition, they report increased difficulty awakening in the morning, heightened mental activity during the night, more frequent and unpleasant dreams, and increased sleepiness during the day (Manber and Armitage 1999).

Incidence

The incidence of episodic insomnia complaints during normal menstruation is essentially unknown. Most women do not specifically complain to their physicians. Between 20% and 40% of women are estimated to have some menstrual-related complaints, which include sleep complaints in many women (Severino and Moline 1995).

Etiology and Pathophysiology

Although hormonal balance clearly can affect sleep, specific correlations between hormone levels and sleep complaints have not proven illuminating. One study showed that women with premenstrual dysphoric disorder have a later onset of melatonin secretion in the luteal phase.

Laboratory Findings

Polysomnographic recordings are not typically necessary; most of these syndromes are identified on the basis of a sleep history that is temporally related to menstruation.

Differential Diagnosis

The physician must consider and rule out other non-menstrual-related sleep disorders.

Treatment

Isolated insomnia complaints during menstruation can be appropriately treated with several nights of a short-acting hypnotic (zolpidem, zaleplon, or a benzodiazepine). Even if each menstrual period is accompanied by only 2 or 3 nights of disturbed sleep, this still means that affected women have impaired sleep for about 10% of their adult lives. There is no reason that these complaints should not be treated symptomatically to prevent the impairments in daytime function associated with several nights of disturbed sleep.

SRIs have been the most commonly used agents to treat the underlying physiological abnormality of premenstrual dysphoric disorder. Other serotonergic antidepressants are second-line agents, and alprazolam and buspirone are considered third-line agents. These drugs often help treat the insomnia complaint that frequently accompanies premenstrual dysphoric disorder (Endicott 2001). If SRIs are used but insomnia persists, adding a benzodiazapine receptor agonist such as zaleplon or zolpidem would be appropriate. Partial sleep deprivation (limiting sleep to 4 hours per night) has also been shown to improve mood symptoms associated with PMS (Parry et al. 1997).

Several cases of premenstrual parasomnia that have been reported appeared to respond to both bedtime self-hypnosis and clonazepam therapy (0.25 mg) (Schenck and Mahowald 1995).

■ SLEEP COMPLAINTS ASSOCIATED WITH MENOPAUSE

One-half to three-quarters of women complain of sleep-onset insomnia, frequent awakenings, and daytime sleepiness during menopause and postmenopause (Baker et al. 1997). Most evidence shows that much of the sleep disturbance is secondary to vasomotor symptoms such as sweats and hot flashes. There is some evidence that some of the sleep disturbance may be the result of a moderately hyperadrenergic state that may accompany the menopausal and postmenopausal period, independent of hot flashes (Freedman 1998).

Estrogen replacement therapy is commonly used to eliminate hot flashes and secondarily improve menopausal sleep. Three of six studies performed in recent years to assess the sleep benefits of estrogen replacement therapy in postmenopausal women found no real change. In studies showing benefit, the most consistent signs of improvement were decreased hot flashes and decreased arousals from sleep, resulting in better sleep continuity and less daytime fatigue (Polo-Kantolo et al. 1999).

Clonidine has also been effectively used to improve sleep and block hot flashes. In women for whom estrogen replacement therapy is contraindicated, clonidine or sedative-hypnotics may be quite effective. Sedative antidepressants such as trazodone can be useful as well. Menopausal women may also be vulnerable to depression or anxiety; assessment and appropriate treatment are warranted.

■ REFERENCES

Altshuler LL, Cohen L Szuba MP, et al: Pharmacologic management of psychiatric illness during pregnancy: dilemmas and guidelines. Am J Psychiatry 153:592–606, 1996

Altshuler LL, Cohen L, Moline M, et al: Expert consensus guidelines for the treatment of depression in women: a new treatment tool. The Economics of Neuroscience 3:48–61, 2001

Ancoli-Israel S, Kripke DF, Mason W: Characteristics of obstructive and central sleep apnea in the elderly: an interim report. Biol Psychiatry 22:741–750, 1987

Baker A, Simpson S, Dawson D: Sleep disruption and mood changes associated with menopause. J Psychosom Res 43:359–369, 1997

Bixler E, Kales A, Soldatos C, et al: Prevalence of sleep disorders: a survey of the Los Angeles metropolitan area. Am J Psychiatry 136:1257–1262, 1979

Campbell SS, Terman M, Lewy AJ, et al: Light treatment for sleep disorders: consensus report, V: age related disturbances. J Biol Rhythms 10:151–154, 1995

Carroll JL, Loughlin GM: Primary snoring in children, in Principles and Practice of Sleep Medicine in the Child. Edited by Ferber R, Kryger M. Philadelphia, PA, WB Saunders, 1995, pp 155–161

Cohen L: Course and treatment of mood disorders during pregnancy and the postpartum period. Paper presented at the annual meeting of the American Psychiatric Association, Chicago, IL, May 2000

Corkum P, Moldofsky H, Hogg-Johnson S: Sleep problems in children with attention-deficit/hyperactivity disorder: impact of subtype, comorbidity, and stimulant medication. J Am Acad Child Adolesc Psychiatry 38:1285–1293, 1999

Dahl RE: Sleep in behavioral and emotional disorders, in Principles and Practice of Sleep Medicine in Children. Edited by Ferber R, Kryger M. Philadelphia, PA, WB Saunders, 1995, pp 147–153

Dahlitz M, Alvarez B, Vignau J, et al: Delayed sleep phase syndrome response to melatonin. Lancet 337:1121–1124, 1991

Davidson-Ward SL, Marcus CL: Obstructive sleep apnea in infants and young children. J Clin Neurophysiol 13:198–207, 1996

Endicott J: Diagnosis and pharmacologic treatment of premenstrual dysphoric disorder. The Economics of Neuroscience 3:44–47, 2001

Ferber R: The sleepless child, in Sleep and Its Disorders in Children. Edited by Guilleminault C. New York, Raven, 1987, pp 141–163

Foley DJ, Monjan AA, Brown SL, et al: Sleep complaints among elderly persons: an epidemiologic study of three communities. Sleep 18:425–432, 1995

Freedman RR: Biochemical, metabolic, and vascular mechanisms in menopausal hot flashes. Fertil Steril 20:332–337, 1998

Goldstein DJ, Corbin LA, Fung MC: Olanzapine-exposed pregnancies and lactation: early experience. J Clin Psychopharmacol 20:394–403, 2000

Gruber R, Sadeh A, Raviv A: Instability of sleep patterns in children with attention-deficit/hyperactivity disorder. J Am Acad Child Adolesc Psychiatry 39:495–501, 2000

Haimov I, Lavie P, Laudon M, et al: Melatonin replacement therapy of elderly insomniacs. Sleep 18:598–603, 1995

Hertz G, Fast V, Feinsilver SH, et al: Sleep in normal late pregnancy. Sleep 15:246–251, 1992

Jan MM: Melatonin for the treatment of handicapped children with severe sleep disorders. Pediatr Neurol 23:229–232, 2000

Kotagal S, Goulding PM: The laboratory assessment of daytime sleepiness in childhood. J Clin Neurophysiol 13:208–218, 1996

Lapierre O, Dumont M: Melatonin treatment of a non-24-hour sleep-wake cycle in a blind retarded child. Biol Psychiatry 38:119–122, 1995

Leger D, Prevot E, Philip P, et al: Sleep disorders in children with blindness. Ann Neurol 46:648–651, 1999

Manber R, Armitage R: Sex, steroids, and sleep: a review. Sleep 22:540–555, 1999

Mark SD, Frank JD: Nocturnal enuresis. Br J Urol 75:427–434, 1995

Mick E, Biederman J, Jetton J, et al: Sleep disturbances associated with attention deficit hyperactivity disorder: the impact of psychiatric comorbidity and pharmacotherapy. J Child Adolesc Psychopharmacol 10:223–231, 2000

Morin CM, Colecchi C, Stone J, et al: Behavioral and pharmacological therapies for late-life insomnia: a randomized controlled trial. JAMA 281:991–999, 1999

Mosko SS, Dickel MJ, Ashorst J: Night to night variability in sleep apnea and sleep-related periodic leg movements in the elderly. Sleep 11:340–348, 1988

Nino-Murcia G, Keenan S: enuresis and sleep, in Sleep and Its Disorders in Children. Edited by Guilleminault C. New York, Raven, 1987, pp 253–267

Owens JA, Maxim R, Nobile C, et al: Parental and self-report of sleep in children with attention- deficit/hyperactivity disorder. Arch Pediatr Adolesc Med 154:549–555, 2000

Parry BL, LeVeau B, Mostofi N, et al: Temperature circadian rhythms during the menstrual cycle and sleep deprivation in premenstrual dysphoric disorder and normal comparison subjects. J Biol Rhythms 12:34–46, 1997

Patten CA, Choi WS, Gillin JC, et al: Depressive symptoms and cigarette smoking predict development and persistence of sleep problems in US adolescents. Pediatrics 106:E23, 2000

Picchietti DL, England SJ, Walters AS, et al: Periodic limb movement disorder and restless legs syndrome in children with attention-deficit hyperactivity disorder. J Child Neurol 13:588–594, 1998

Polo-Kantolo P, Erkkola R, Irjala K, et al: Effect of short-term transdermal estrogen replacement therapy on sleep: a randomized, double-blind crossover trial in postmenopausal women. Fertil Steril 71:873–880, 1999

Prinz PN: Sleep and sleep disorders in older adults. J Clin Neurophysiol 12:139–146, 1995

Reynolds CF, Soloff PH, Kupfer DJ, et al: Depression in borderline patients: a prospective EEG study. Psychiatry Res 14:1–15, 1985

Schenck CH, Mahowald MW: Two cases of premenstrual sleep terrors and injurious sleep-walking. J Psychosom Obstet Gynaecol 16:79–84, 1995

Schweiger MS: Sleep disturbances in pregnancy. Am J Obstet Gynecol 114:879–882, 1972

Severino SK, Moline ML: Premenstrual syndrome. Drugs 49:71–82, 1995

Thorpy MJ, Korman E, Spielman AJ: Delayed sleep phase syndrome in adolescents. Journal of Adolescent Health Care 9:22–27, 1988

Tobias NE: Management of nocturnal enuresis. Nurs Clin North Am 35:37–60, 2000

Van Cauter E, Leproult R, Plat L: Age related changes in slow wave sleep and REM sleep and relationship with growth hormone and cortisol in healthy men. JAMA 284:861–868, 2000

Weissbluth M: Sleep and the colicky infant, in Sleep and Its Disorders in Children. Edited by Guilleminault C. New York, Raven, 1987, pp 129–140

Wiggs L: Sleep problems in children with developmental disorders. J R Soc Med 94:177–179, 2001

Wisner KL, Perel JM, Blumer J: Serum sertraline and *N*-desmethylsertraline levels in breast-feeding mother-infant pairs. Am J Psychiatry 155:690–692, 1998

INDEX

*Page numbers printed in **boldface** type refer to tables or figures.*